A Place Called Self

A Place Called Self

A COMPANION WORKBOOK

Women, Sobriety, and
Radical Transformation

Stephanie Brown, Ph.D.

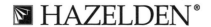 HAZELDEN®

Hazelden
Center City, Minnesota 55012-0176
1-800-328-0094
1-651-213-4590 (Fax)
www.hazelden.org
© 2006 by Hazelden Foundation

Library of Congress Cataloging-in-Publication Data

Brown, Stephanie, 1944–
    A place called self : women, sobriety, and radical transformation : a companion
workbook / Stephanie Brown.
      p. cm.
    ISBN-13: 978-1-59285-355-7
    ISBN-10: 1-59285-355-2
    1. Recovering alcoholics—Psychology—Problems, exercises, etc. 2. Women
alcoholics—Psychology—Problems, exercises, etc. 3. Alcoholics—Rehabilitation—
Problems, exercises, etc. I. Title.

HV5275.B76 2006
616.86'103—dc22
                                                                                            2006041201

10 09 08 07 06   6 5 4 3 2 1

Cover design by Theresa Gedig
Interior design by Rachel Holscher
Typesetting by Stanton Publication Services, Inc.

For all women in recovery
and, as always, for Makenzie

Contents

Acknowledgments

My life is about gratitude: deep, wide, soul-embracing gratitude. I have been helped directly by so many people who have passed on to me their "experience, strength, and hope" over many years. I have been helped and supported in my personal journey and on my professional path to ask and answer difficult questions about addiction and recovery. Throughout my journey on these interwoven paths, I have lived the paradoxes of recovery that I now write about. I have faced them and found them in my own experience. I have gained strength and hope through finding the power in powerlessness and the wisdom to know the deep truth of "alone-together."

And so I say thank you to all who have helped me, supported me, and shown me the way.

A big part of this journey is digging deep. And so, in this workbook for *A Place Called Self,* I encourage women who are still drinking and actively addicted in other ways to dig deep; ask yourselves the tough questions and stand by to learn the answers. I encourage women in recovery to do exactly the same thing: ask yourselves the tough questions, dig deeper, and see who's there. Being in recovery is a journey of finding your self. This workbook can guide you in looking inward to deepen and strengthen your recovery.

Thank you to the countless women and men who have shared their recoveries with me as friends, colleagues, and clients. Thanks to all my colleagues over the years for support in carrying a new message about what happens in recovery. Thanks to Hazelden—a strong pillar of addiction treatment and a strong publishing team. Thank you, Becky Post, for being a wonderful editor: a great teacher with a keen sensitivity to what women need, and the skills to provide it.

As always, I'm deeply grateful to my husband, Bob Harris, and our daughter, Makenzie, for our loving family.

Introduction

Welcome to recovery. In this workbook you and I will continue the journey that we began in my book *A Place Called Self: Women, Sobriety, and Radical Transformation.* We will start by remembering our active addictions, "what it was like" to lose control, and how it felt to shift into abstinence. We will remember that first experience of being dry, of being without alcohol or our other drugs of choice, and we will remember the long, hard, and infinitely rewarding path of recovery, a path of finding the real you. This book is about getting in touch with the true you, the woman deep inside who's always been there, but who disappeared into the false self of addiction. The real you is the woman you will find by being in recovery and engaging in a developmental process of healthy growth.

In this workbook you will compare your experiences in recovery to infant and child development. As you reflect on your old life and your new life, you will see that growing up all over again in recovery is similar to growing up for the first time. There's no doubt about it, growing up again is incredibly hard. It is painful and scary to feel so vulnerable, to not know what to do. But soon, you will know what to do, and you will also feel hopeful and even excited. With stable abstinence, you will experience a new safety and the thrill of new learning without your drugs or addictive behaviors. Soon you will experience the promise of finding your self—the real, true you. And this may be a person you've never known before.

This workbook is your guide, no matter where you are in your recovery. You may have brand new sobriety or many months or years. Maybe you are still drinking/using or you have recently relapsed. No matter where you are, you can locate yourself on this path.

Step by tiny step, we will take this journey together, through the stages of active addiction and the developmental process called recovery. You will learn what happens, what it takes to be in recovery, and you will see that none of this makes common sense.

You're on a path, I'm on a path, and it is a path full of myths and paradoxes.

Quite simply, recovery is not what you think it is. You will be surprised all along the journey at the new ways you see yourself and the world. Recovery is not simple; it is not a straight line. You don't go from A to B to C. There are detours, mudflats, rocky points, and flat easy spaces on this recovery journey. Just like normal child development, healthy recovery growth has its ups and downs, ins and outs. You'll stumble now and then and you'll move easily at other times. No matter how hard, or how easy it is, you learn to stay on this path.

This workbook is your personal journal, your guide to deepening your recovery development. It is not the same as working the Twelve Steps of Alcoholics Anonymous (AA) or other Twelve Step programs. And it shouldn't be a replacement. My books are designed to be complementary to the Twelve Steps, to enhance and deepen your self-exploration.

The chapters in this workbook follow the chapters in *A Place Called Self*, summarizing the major points, offering questions to think about, and making suggestions for writing. The exercises are designed to help you think about your self in new ways. First you will look at how you lost your self, your real self, to addiction. You are going to remember your actions, your thoughts, and your feelings. Then you will examine these same things as you proceed through the stages of recovery. By being active and engaging in these exercises, you will find the real you.

Is this a hard process? Yes. Is it worth it? I believe deeply that it is worth it. I've been on this recovery road for thirty-four years and I continue to be awed by what I learn. To proceed, take it slowly. Let the descriptions and exercises sink in. Try doing an exercise today, put it aside, and look it over tomorrow. Add to it, take away. It's all about you. It's your story, your life. You will be going from false to real, all the way through. If you get scared or stumped, or if you feel overwhelmed, take a time-out. Stay on the recovery road, increase your meetings, and perhaps seek professional help. Then, as you feel calm and your sense of security returns, pick up your deepening process again. At the end of each chapter I will ask you to think about the following questions: What is real for me now? What am I learning? How do I think about myself and about others now? And I will also ask: What is the gift you recognize today? What is healthy recovery? Who are you?

The gifts, full of paradox and perhaps hard to see, will accumulate as you find and grow your healthy self.

Welcome to recovery.

PART ONE

Welcome to Recovery

What Is Recovery?

This book is about recovery from addiction. So let's start by defining addiction. Simply put, addiction is the loss of control. It is the inability to stop drinking, using other drugs, eating, gambling, or acting out other behaviors once you've started. But addiction is more than behavior. It starts with an emotional attachment. A woman forms an emotional bond to alcohol, a prescription medicine, food, or even another person; this bond becomes a compulsive attachment that she can't do without. The object of her addiction becomes her best friend, her lover, and the demon that will destroy her. Addiction becomes a deep loss of self.

On the other hand, you may think that the definition of recovery is simply not drinking, not using, not eating too much or too little, or not spending money all the time. You may think that recovery is the same thing as being abstinent. It's not. Becoming abstinent is an event. Recovery is a long-term *developmental process* that follows the event. It is not a quick fix.

Myths of Recovery

You may also think that recovery means you are well and doing everything right. This is one of the great myths about recovery: You were *bad* when you were drinking/using, and you will be *good* when you are sober. Recovery is not going from bad to good. It has nothing to do with bad or good. You will learn that recovery is going from false to real. It is about letting go of the false self of your addiction and finding your real self.

Additionally, you may have hoped that once you started recovery you would stop being dependent (if you ever really recognized that your addiction was a dependency). You may have envisioned a new, sober you, a woman who was self-sufficient, a woman who didn't need anybody or anything. Well, this is not the way it goes either. It is another myth. You will move from your unhealthy dependence on your substance or addictive behavior to a new, healthy dependence on others in recovery. This is truly baffling at first, but it is the foundation for healthy growth in recovery.

Recovery is not a reversal or a restoration of self. It is not going from bad to good or from dependent to self-sufficient. Recovery is so much more. Recovery is a process of radical growth and change, which often includes a deep transformation of the self. Recovery thus becomes the development of a new self.

Paradoxes of Recovery

As you enter recovery and follow this path toward a new self, you will discover new truths—new ideas and new ways of thinking about yourself. Your new foundation of self is grounded in paradox. What happens in recovery doesn't make sense to the old, false you of your addiction.

We will cover all the paradoxes in more detail later in this workbook, but for now let's name the two that form the core of the new process of recovery:

1. We are powerless—that's what loss of control is—and we are responsible for being powerless.
2. We all need others on whom we can depend, but we are ultimately alone. This is the spirituality of recovery, the knowledge that we have a basic need for others.

In the following exercises, let's think about your definitions of addiction and recovery, the myths you may have held, and your understanding of paradox.

Exercises: Thinking about Addiction, Recovery, and My Self

Many people think that addiction means losing control. It really means that a person can't stop drinking or using other drugs once she starts, or she can't stop eating once she reaches for that dessert or other binge food.

- How do I define addiction?

_____

_____

_____

_____

_____

Many women believe that being addicted means they failed because they lost control of their lives. They realize that they failed to be good mothers, or good wives or partners, or good workers. These are such painful issues to face that many women say, "I can't be addicted. It can't be true of me. I can't bear to face this failure." What was it like for you?

- When you were still actively addicted, what did it mean to you if you thought you might be addicted?

_____

_____

_____

_____

_____

_____

_____

It is normal for a woman to tell herself that she is not addicted. She can easily make excuses for why she needs to drink, take addictive medication, or nibble away. She will explain why her need to drink, to use, to eat, or to spend is not an addiction; why she's not out of control. And so the cycle goes.

- During your active addiction, how did you explain to yourself that you had not lost control? That you were not an alcoholic? That you were not addicted? What was your story?

_____

_____

_____

_____

_____

_____

_____

Addiction is more than behavior. It is more than the loss of control. A woman forms a deep, intense emotional bond with her addictive object (her substance or behavior). It is this emotional attachment—the intense craving and need to have her drug—that drives her repeated behavior and leads to the loss of her self. Let's think about your attachment to your drug.

- How was your addiction an emotional attachment? Describe how you felt about your drug or your addictive behavior. *Who* was it? *What* was it? How did it *work?*

_____

_____

_____

_____

_____

During active addiction, many women believe that recovery will take them from *bad* to *good* and from being *dependent* to being *self-sufficient.* They want to become strong, not weak, and they believe that they won't need anybody or anything to help them. Some women have a grim mental picture of recovery: an image of sheer deprivation and desperation. Other women believe they will be lost without their "best friend" (their addictive substance or behavior). What about you? What *myths* did you have about recovery?

- What did you think recovery would be like? How did you define recovery when you were still actively addicted? What myths did you believe about recovery?

_____

_____

_____

_____

_____

• How do you think about recovery now? What is recovery?

_____

_____

_____

_____

_____

You know by now that becoming abstinent is the event and recovery is a process. Recovery is not magic and it doesn't happen quickly. You have to be engaged; you have to be active, and then you will grow into your healthy self. Think about what the word *process* means for you.

• How is recovery a process for you? What does that mean?

_____

_____

_____

_____

_____

The developmental process of recovery is grounded on paradox. Paradox turns things around; what was old and false in your active addiction becomes the source for freedom and healthy, positive growth in recovery. Understanding paradox gives you a new way of seeing and thinking about your self.

• What is powerlessness? How did you think about being powerless when you were actively addicted? How do you think about being powerless now?

_____

_____

_____

_____

_____

- What is responsibility? How did you think about responsibility when you were actively addicted? How do you think about responsibility now?

  _____

  _____

  _____

  _____

  _____

- Describe how you can be both powerless and responsible at the same time. What does this paradox mean for you? How does this paradox work for you?

  _____

  _____

  _____

  _____

  _____

- How are you dependent on others? How do you need others? In what ways are you self-reliant?

  _____

  _____

  _____

  _____

  _____

Many women in recovery experience a sense of transformation. Sometimes it is felt right away with new abstinence and sometimes not until long into recovery. The transformation involves going from false to real. And it involves asking for help. Now, at the beginning of your recovery journey, let's think about transformation.

- After you became abstinent, did you experience a transformation? What happened?

_____

_____

_____

_____

_____

What Is Real?

As we get ready to journey through the stages of recovery, let's think about *what is real*. Wherever you are in your personal recovery development, what is real for you today?

- What does real mean for you today? What do you know absolutely? What is true? If you wish, think back to when you were actively addicted. What was real then? What did your world look like? What did you believe?

_____

_____

_____

_____

_____

_____

_____

_____

_____

_____

_____

What Is the Gift?

Whether your day is hard, rocky, painful, or smooth and soft, recovery does bring gifts—such as improved relationships or improved health. What gifts do you feel most strongly about now?

- Name some gifts in your life and how they improve your life.

_____

_____

_____

_____

_____

_____

- Name some benefits of recovery that you have yet to realize.

_____

_____

_____

_____

_____

_____

- Name some gifts of recovery that you desire, but understand that acquiring them is beyond your control or will.

_____

_____

_____

_____

_____

PART TWO

A Developmental Process

Finding "a place called self" in recovery is a developmental process. Development usually means forward growth, movement that builds in layers and stages. And that is exactly what healthy growth in recovery is: forward development, growing up again. But it is not just one straight line moving ahead. In recovery, development is forward, backward, sideways, upside down, and inside out. It is a long, hard road of fits and starts, with a steady underlying forward flow.

Being addicted is backward development. It is like an undertow that pulls you down and under, until you are not moving forward at all. This kind of backward development involves increasing loss of control. A woman becomes dependent on her addiction to take care of her and eventually her dependence harms her instead. She is stuck at the bottom, in a cage; or she is trying to go up the down escalator. She can't stop, she can't get out, she can't get off.

A woman relinquishes her self as she becomes addicted. She gives up what she knows of her real self and begins to build a false self. Being addicted becomes an ongoing process of backward development, of shutting down and shutting off what is real. Turning this backward slide around is the heart of recovery.

The woman at the bottom comes face-to-face with herself. She sees, for a brief instant, that she is trapped, that she has lost control to her unhealthy dependence. If she can hold on to this new truth, she can begin a recovery process. After having given up her self, she will now begin to reclaim that self and to build a new self.

Recovery development occurs in stages that parallel, metaphorically, human development, from infant to toddler to adolescent to adult. We will follow these stages, looking first at the backward development of addiction, and then exploring how the woman makes her separation from her drug of choice and from her active addiction. This separation sets in motion a new development of self. Recovery development is the birth and growth of a healthy self.

Exercises: Thinking about Addiction as a Developmental Process

Recovery from active addiction involves the growth of a new self. It is analogous to infant and child development, a process of normal growth that has clear tasks and defined stages over many years.

- Has your recovery been a developmental process so far? How?

_____

_____

_____

_____

_____

- Can you remember key events or milestones for you in your recovery growth? What are they?

_____

_____

_____

_____

_____

• Do you remember feeling like an infant or a young child during new recovery? What was it like?

_____

_____

_____

_____

• Did you have periods of feeling like an adolescent? What was it like?

_____

_____

_____

_____

• Where are you in your recovery development now? Do you feel grown up? Do you have a new self, a new you?

_____

_____

_____

_____

• Who are you now?

_____

_____

_____

_____

Losing a Self

THE ACTIVE ADDICTION STAGE

Addiction means the loss of control. It means you can't predictably stop drinking, using, eating, spending, or gambling once you've started. Being addicted also usually means that you tell yourself you are fine. You tell yourself all the reasons why you don't have a problem. Then you explain why you *need* to drink this much, take all these pills, nibble all day long, spend too much, or gamble away your savings. You explain exactly why you *need* your addiction in a way that lets you keep right on going. So, you deny and explain in order to maintain. That's it, a vicious circle.

As you get caught in this downward spiral, this backward development, you lose more than the control of your drinking, drugging, or other addictive behavior. You lose your self, the true, real you that is now buried deep inside, under the lies of your addiction. You begin to create a false self, a false front, like a movie set, a cardboard screen around the real you. This new, false you is built on your denial, your distortion, and all your false explanations for why you're fine. You are hooked, now tightly bound to your substance or your compulsive behavior. You tell yourself: "I am not an alcoholic/addict. I can control my drinking/using." These two beliefs form the core of your shaky foundation. It's like quicksand, pulling you down.

As you become more and more out of control, you need to strengthen your *defenses*, the distortions in the way you see, feel, and think that keep you pretending and cut off from yourself. You need the substance to feel okay, but if you admit you need the substance, you can't feel okay about yourself. You're caught in a terrible bind, so caught that you ultimately shut down your deepest experience of self.

Why Women Become Addicted

Asking "why" may not be a good idea if you are still active in your addiction. You are likely to tell yourself why you are not addicted, rather than seriously consider why and how you got to where you are. But, if you are in recovery and looking back, asking "why" is a good idea.

You will do this automatically as you begin to work the Twelve Steps of AA or another program. Looking at who you were and what happened to you as you lost control are central to the work of recovery.

As women reflect back, most conclude that drinking or using other drugs was initially a positive experience. It helped them cope or filled a gaping hole within. Perhaps drinking got them going. It was the energizer that fueled a good feeling or mood. Or, popping a little pill gave them the illusion that they could control some problematic aspect of life. They could cover up, fit in, or fade away. Whatever they needed right then, the pill would do the job. Some women use food as a reward. Or they spend to reduce their stress. Whatever the reason, whatever the *need,* there's something to drink or pop or do to take control. Trouble is, loss of control is just around the bend.

The Process of Becoming Addicted

The process of becoming addicted is different than the "whys." It is the "turn toward" alcohol, or pills, or whatever else will fill the need. The process is the actual experience of beginning to *need* more of the addictive substance or behavior to quiet your anxiety or cravings. As you begin to feel your loss of control, along with the panic of your *need,* you bolster your defenses to prove that nothing is wrong. Becoming addicted is the loss of your self. You bury your real, true self beneath the facade of your false sense of control.

Addiction and Trauma

Trauma literally means injury. Whether that injury is physical or emotional, it can leave a woman feeling helpless. Many women who have experienced trauma at the hands of others turn to alcohol or other drugs to cope with their feelings and victimization.

But these women also lose control to the power of their addiction. Being addicted can be a trauma in itself. Active addiction is the state of helplessness that comes with the loss of control. It is the reality that the woman works so hard to deny as she sinks deeper into isolation and despair. The addicted woman lives in a state of chronic self-inflicted trauma.

It is almost always difficult and painful to recognize that her efforts to cope are causing her even more despair. As she comes face to face with this reality she "gets ready" for recovery. She comes to see, "I am an alcoholic/addict. I have lost control." As she experiences defeat in all her efforts to gain control, she asks for help and learns she can't "do" recovery alone.

❧

Exercises: My Addiction and the Loss of My Self

What Was It Like?

Addiction is all about control and the loss of control. Most people believe that self-control is a virtue and that being in control equals being powerful. So recognizing the loss of control feels like a terrible failure. Ironically, no human being has total control, yet seeing this reality is threatening. People expend great energy to prove that there are no limits to the power they hold. It is a great fallacy and the core of the addictive cycle. Women keep trying to "get control," only to lose it and try again. The end of this vicious cycle doesn't come until she accepts her loss of control and her inability to regain it.

- What did you used to think about control? How did you explain to yourself that you were in control?

_____

_____

_____

_____

- What do you think about control now?

_____

_____

_____

_____

- What was it like to lose control? Describe your experience or write a story about a woman who lost control. What was it like for you/her? What happened?

_____

_____

_____

_____

- List five things you still believe you should be able to control. What is it you can't stop doing now? What is it you can't see about yourself now? What is it you can't know?

_____

_____

_____

_____

_____

What Did It Mean?

Both men and women experience loss of control. Men and women interpret loss of control in different ways. Men tend to see the loss of control as a failure of masculine competitiveness, a failure in male power. Some women see their loss of control in the same way. But almost all women also see their loss of control as a failure in relationships. Losing control means that they have failed as wives, partners, and mothers. Accepting your loss of control is an acceptance of limits to self-sufficiency and of the fundamental need for help outside of the self.

- What did it mean to you to lose control when you were actively addicted?

_____

_____

_____

_____

_____

- What does it mean now?

_____

_____

_____

_____

_____

- How do you feel about limits? List five ways you know you are limited now.

- What does it mean to you to ask for help? What does it feel like?

What Is Unhealthy Dependence?

Most people believe that dependence is a bad thing. People consider *need* to be a bad word. They want to be self-sufficient and not rely on others. And so, you made your "turn toward" alcohol or other drugs as a way of meeting your needs, a way of not needing anybody or anything. You developed your unhealthy bond to alcohol, other drugs, food, shopping, or gambling as a way to cope, to take care of yourself. And it turned on you.

- What was your "turn toward" alcohol or your "turn toward" addiction? Do you remember crossing a line or sealing your emotional attachment to an addictive substance or behavior?

- What was it like to be dependent on your substance or addictive behavior? Write a paragraph describing your dependency during your active addiction.

_____

_____

_____

_____

- What does craving feel like? Describe the experience, past or present, or just list words that come to mind.

_____

_____

_____

_____

Addiction and Trauma

A woman who has experienced trauma often cannot maintain a healthy sense of self or connection to others. Trauma involves intense feelings of helplessness, fear, loss of control, and a threat of annihilation of the self. Being addicted involves this kind of loss of control. Being addicted is the state of being overwhelmed and unable to maintain or restore internal order. It is precisely this reality of trauma that women and men will work the hardest to deny. Nobody wants to feel this much threat and this much loss of control. So people work hard to say it isn't true.

- How was your addiction traumatic for you?

_____

_____

_____

_____

- Does being in recovery ever feel traumatic?

_____

_____

_____

_____

- What traumas have you experienced in your life? As you feel ready, at any point in your recovery, write your stories of what happened What were the events, who were the people, and what was it like to feel threatened, unsafe, endangered? These are difficult questions that take time to answer. You may want to work with your sponsor, a therapist, or perhaps a clergyperson as you delve into remembering the painful experiences of loss of control in your life.

_____

_____

_____

_____

What Is Real?

- As you remember back to your active addiction, and as you think about what it was like to lose control, ask now, what does _real_ mean for you today? What do you know absolutely? What is true? What is real today?

_____

_____

_____

_____

_____

What Is the Gift?

- You have been through the past, you have remembered and you have accepted what is real. What is your gift of recovery today? What can you feel, see, or know about you or your recovery that you couldn't recognize before? Or, what is it that you feel deeply and strongly again right now? What is your gift of seeing and knowing once again?

∽ Chapter Three ∞

Recovery Shock

THE TRANSITION STAGE

Recovery means you are no longer drinking, using drugs, or engaged in other compulsive behaviors. You are abstinent, but recovery is more than being dry. Recovery means you are actively engaged in a process of new development. It means you are finding your new self, the woman who recognizes that she lost control. Being in recovery means you now know "I am an alcoholic/addict. I cannot control my drinking/using."

Surrender and New Attachment

You reached the end of your active addiction when you couldn't do it anymore, when you saw that you couldn't stop and you knew you needed help. You gave up believing that you'd get control, if only you could figure out the magic answer. This painful experience of surrender, of accepting defeat, opened the path for you to move into recovery. You gave up your attachment to your drug and found a new caring attachment in recovery. You allowed yourself to invest in AA, Al-Anon, Overeaters Anonymous (OA), Narcotics Anonymous (NA), or another Twelve Step program. Hopefully, you turned to other women in recovery.

You switched your deep need, your dependency on addictive substances and behavior, for a deep dependency on AA or another Twelve Step program and women in recovery. You did not stop needing. You did not suddenly become self-sufficient. You just changed the way you fill that need. You went from the bottle or the pill to the meetings and the people of recovery.

Recovery Shock

You probably hoped that stopping your active addiction would give you peace and a sense of control. What a shock to find that you could feel just as out of control as ever. You had no idea you'd wake up in new abstinence to find that you don't know anything about how to live in healthy ways. You don't know who you are. You don't know what it is you don't know. This can be a frightening jolt, a terrifying shock. Why? Here's where new development comes in.

A Developmental Process

The challenges of early recovery are similar to growing up all over again. You may feel like an infant with raw and primitive emotions. You're a bundle of instincts. You may even feel like screaming. You sometimes feel like you need the nurturance of your mother.

Just like a newborn, your first task is to reach out for help. You reach for a mother substitute. You find AA and settle in to make an attachment to this nurturing and supportive source of help. Then, in the context of this new dependence, you begin a new process of development.

Behavior First

When an infant seeks a response from her parents or primary caregivers, she is seeking comfort and security. A woman in early recovery similarly seeks comfort and reassurance. Her job in new recovery is to focus on new behavior. She learns immediately to act quickly on her cravings and impulses, reaching out to a new source of soothing. It is in a phone call, a meeting, or reading the literature of recovery. She learns to tolerate her discomfort as she learns to trust that her anxieties will subside. She learns to wait out an intense craving by turning to recovery behavior. The craving will subside.

Head Learning

As she learns the new behaviors of abstinence, the woman in early recovery also listens. She identifies with other women who are on this recovery path and she begins to take in new knowledge about herself: who she was and what she did when she was active in her addiction and who she is now. She begins to know her true story and to tell it. Through this process of being abstinent and identifying with other women in recovery, she begins to find her real self, the self that she buried under the cover of her addiction. She finds that being in recovery is all about reality. It is all about being real.

Heart Learning

Throughout this new process of recovery, you will begin to feel. Sometimes the feelings come right away, just as soon as you've had your last drink. That can be a lot to tolerate.

Or, the feelings may remain frozen for a while. You may not feel anything right away except the newness of being dry and perhaps even the excitement of this new world. When your emotions come, you reach out again, no matter when this happens. If it is early on, you may need a lot of extra support. You go to many meetings and perhaps seek professional help. You build your recovery foundation, and use your program to deal with your emotions as they arise.

Feelings may frighten you at first. They can be painful. That's why you drank or used all kinds of addictive behaviors to quiet them. Now, you tolerate feelings and go to work to understand them. Feelings also reflect the reality of the past and present. Whether your feelings are negative or positive, they can be frightening. Without the numbing effects of alcohol, drugs, or addictive activities, emotions can be very intense. Understanding all of your feelings will be an important part of your recovery work in the months and years ahead.

A Focus on Self

You know by now that recovery is all about finding and focusing on your "self." This is, of course, paradoxical, if you always tried to be the best woman you could—in service to others. Putting your self first was selfish. So how do you ever get it that you must find your own true self? It is through this new dependence you've found. By listening to others you will learn what is true for you. You will find the boundaries of your separate self through others.

Recovery and Trauma

In the past you lost control of yourself. You may also have lost control to someone else. You may have been the victim of someone else's out-of-control behavior, abuse, and violence. As a child, you may have been molested by a trusted adult. You may have lived with trauma, the experience of being hurt, helpless, and out of control. These memories and the feelings of terror that went with them will come to you sooner or later in recovery. You will know them, remember and deal with them when they surface. It's not easy. It's an axiom of recovery: *You may feel worse rather than better during new recovery*. You'll learn to repeatedly ask yourself, "Is the pain I'm feeling a warning of relapse? Am I about to drink or use, or is this pain a part of normal recovery growth?"

Often you can't tell the difference between pain that may cause a relapse and pain that is a normal part of recovery. So you keep solid in your recovery program. You maintain your behaviors of abstinence, you listen and identify, and you work the Twelve Steps. As you proceed, you may seek professional help to add to your understanding and to help you sort out which pain is normal pain and which may cause a relapse.

✣

Exercises: Recovery Shock

What Happened?

New recovery is a shock. But so is getting there. Most women have an experience of hitting bottom. They come to a deep clarity that they have lost control.

- As you came to the end of your drinking or using, what happened?

- Did you hit bottom? What was it like? Describe what happened to lead you to surrender.

New Attachment

- After you quit drinking (or using drugs or another addictive behavior), did you reach out for help? Describe your "turn toward recovery." Did you make a call? Did you go to a Twelve Step meeting? How did you make a connection to something or someone involved with recovery?

- Describe how you felt during your first days of recovery. Could you feel a new bond with AA or with people in recovery? A treatment center? A therapist? Your physician? Your minister or rabbi? Could you feel a sense of safety, a sense of trust that there was someone or something to reach out to? Or, was it difficult to trust, to reach out? Did you move back and forth from drinking/ using to abstinence and back again? What is your story of your journey into recovery?

_____

_____

_____

_____

_____

Recovery Shock and New Development

It is hard to wake up to the reality of not knowing what to do next. You stopped drinking/using, but now what? It is like the shock of ice water when you realize you don't know how to *not drink* or *not use*. You knew how to tell yourself that you should stop, and you knew how to tell yourself that you would stop, but you don't actually know how to stop and stay stopped. Once again, welcome to recovery. You are like an infant who must depend on someone else for her survival. You have to reach out too. You will be like an infant for a while as you allow yourself to depend on the care of other people in recovery. Hopefully you will feel held by the support around you. When you begin to learn the behaviors of abstinence, you are on your way to growing up again.

Behavioral Learning

- What new behaviors of recovery did you learn immediately? List the behaviors that worked for you. What behaviors do you suggest to others who are new?

_____

_____

_____

_____

_____

• What did you do when you had a craving? How did you learn to tolerate discomfort? What do you do now when you feel discomfort?

_____

_____

_____

_____

_____

Head Learning

• Can you remember your first experience of identifying with someone else in recovery? Of knowing that this person had been there; that she or he knew what it was like? Who was that person? Describe your experience of feeling that bond of identification.

_____

_____

_____

_____

_____

• Can you remember beginning to listen? What was it like to take in the words of others in recovery? What did you hear? Was it hard to listen? Easy? Describe your early days of learning the new words of recovery. Just like a toddler learning to talk, what was it like for you?

_____

_____

_____

_____

_____

Heart Learning

- Can you remember your first feeling in new abstinence? What was it? Describe that first feeling and what you did with it.

- Describe what it was like for you to begin to feel in recovery. What feelings did you have and how did you work with them?

- Do you have a "feeling story" of recovery? What happened and what is it like now?

A Focus on Self

Paying attention to your self is one of the hardest tasks in recovery. At first you have no idea how to do this. You question yourself, but answer about somebody else. Each time you try to think about you—who you are, what you did, what you felt—you describe someone else. It is too hard to claim your self and to begin to know who you are.

But that's exactly what you will do in recovery. You will begin to recognize your self. You will begin to make active choices on your behalf. You will begin to learn recovery behavior, language, and feelings.

- What was it like to focus on your self? Could you do it? What could you see about you? Did you automatically focus on others? Describe the process of how you came to have a story. How does your story continue to unfold?

_____

_____

_____

_____

_____

Recovery and Trauma

You know trauma. You know what it is like to feel completely helpless. You have been there. Now you may remember, all too soon, as the feelings flood you in new recovery. Or you will remember slowly over time. But you will remember and you will feel. Your task is to stay in recovery. Use all of your recovery knowledge, your new program tools, to keep you grounded.

Also remember that you may not be able to tell the difference: Do your intense feelings or cravings to drink or use mean you're about to relapse, or are they a sign that you're working hard in recovery? If you stay on the path, you will know in time.

- Continue to think about trauma, following the exercises in chapter 2. How was your addiction traumatic for you?

_____

_____

_____

_____

- Does being in recovery ever feel traumatic? How?

- What recovery tools work best for you when you feel overwhelmed, scared, or on shaky recovery ground?

- What traumas have you experienced in your life? As you feel ready, at any point in your recovery, begin to write your stories of what happened. What were the events, who were the people involved, and what was it like to feel threatened, unsafe, endangered? These are difficult questions that take time. You may want to work with your sponsor, a therapist, or perhaps a clergy-person as you delve into remembering the painful experiences of loss of control in your life.

What Is Real?

- As you think about new abstinence and recovery shock, what is real today? What do you know absolutely? What is true?

_____

_____

_____

_____

_____

_____

_____

What Is the Gift?

You have been through the beginning of recovery, you have felt the shock, and you are staying abstinent one step at a time. You have made an attachment to AA or another source of help, and you are in the infantile state of new growth. You are learning new behaviors, words, and feelings, and you are growing into knowing who you are.

- What is your gift today? What can you feel, see, or know about you or your recovery that you couldn't recognize before?

_____

_____

_____

_____

_____

The Growth of a New Self

THE EARLY RECOVERY STAGE

You likely recall what craving felt like. You were driven by that intensity within, the revving up, the need to do something—anything—quickly to quiet down, calm down. Once you made contact with the substance of your choice, you could sigh and relax. But the sense of relief was always temporary. Now you know that recovery allows you to exhale and experience long-standing relief. You can take a breath and trust that you won't suddenly reach for the bottle. Or worse, find the glass close to your lips.

Early Recovery Is Safe and Stable

Early recovery brings a feeling of safety. You are no longer driven by impulse. You no longer need to be in recovery action every minute to protect yourself from drinking (or using drugs or another addictive behavior). You are anchored in recovery. You have roots and you have a solid foundation of recovery development. You are no longer a squealing ball of infant instinct. Now you are a toddler, a preschooler, and you are off to elementary school. Early recovery is a long period of active learning: strengthening recovery behavior, building your new identity as an alcoholic or addicted woman, and opening up to feelings.

Recovery Learning

Early recovery development is still step-by-step, inch-by-inch. It is a building-block process. You may occasionally feel frustrated or scared and want to forget the past or skip the incremental steps of recovery work. Try to resist this call to leapfrog to a higher level. If you miss the day-to-day process of learning to focus on you, of remembering the past, and of assessing who you are and where you are in the present, you may end up with holes in your recovery development. Just like a growing child who misses critical developmental tasks, you too may begin to feel that you are playing catch-up. Something is missing.

Early recovery is all about reality, about finding your real self. It is a process of discovery and building, not a one-time event. You continue to pay attention and to strengthen your recovery behavior. Now you are able to dig in, to ask yourself hard questions such as "What did I do?" and "What happened?" As your recovery language grows, you will learn more about you. As you put words to old behavior, thoughts, and feelings, they become real. Language helps to quiet the intensity of your feelings. Soon, you will be telling your story. As you speak about yourself, you strengthen your bond to others. You build connections. You are coming to know yourself through listening to others. Now you share yourself to be known by others.

Relationships

As you move through the months and years of early recovery, you now can look outward. Your sense of your recovering self is getting stronger, and you won't get lost by focusing on others. You can now begin to think about your relationships. You will likely start this process as you reach the Fourth Step. Looking closely at yourself will also bring other people into your world of exploration. You explore your past beliefs and patterns of relating, and you apply your program of recovery to your closest relationships.

Dealing with Emotion

Recovery behavior, thinking, and language will help you open up your feelings. You can now make sense of your emotions—positive and negative—and you can let them out without fearing that you will lose control and never get it back.

Most people think it is the negative feelings that will threaten you in recovery. But often, especially for women, it is the positive feelings. Women are often afraid to feel good. Feeling good means feeling guilty. Or frightened. Feeling bad is a lot more familiar.

Growth Hurdles

The woman in recovery faces growth hurdles all along the way. She longs for intimacy, but fears it; she longs to feel her own strong self, yet she feels anxious about being separate and responsible. She may feel intense shame for what she did or did not do throughout her life. And she may feel a strong undertow to go back to drinking/using, to stop all this recovery nonsense, this growth of her self.

Staying on the Path

How do you stay in recovery? How do you do this hard work of development? First, you must maintain your attachment to recovery and follow the Twelve Step map. You now know yourself alone and you know yourself through relationships. You have been alone and alone-together the whole time. You are developing your power through a "Higher" Other, rather than depending on you alone, or looking to other people to do it for you.

Recovery and Trauma

Now comes the hardest work. You remember the past and you acknowledge the realities of the present. You become accountable. The remembering may be painful, but you can take it slowly. What happened? What did you do? How did you lose control? Were you the victim of someone else's loss of control, violence, abuse, molestation? Were you the abuser? It is incredibly hard to see clearly. In fact, things may never be clear. They are complicated, layered, and confusing, but recovery shows us how to stay focused on the path of self-awareness, self-knowing, and telling the truth.

Relapse

If you have established a solid, stable early recovery, relapse is less likely. You have the tools and you know how to use them. But is relapse possible? Yes, it is always possible. You continue to pay attention to basic recovery behavior and principles. You stay close to your program and your mentors—the women who teach you and challenge you. You continue to look inward, to question yourself. As you stay sober in early recovery, you are developing a capacity to be honest.

You watch for holes in your recovery development. You work the Steps. You question yourself. And you remember the recovery axiom: *Is the pain I'm feeling a sign of healthy growth or a warning of relapse?* When you can't tell the answer, which may be often, you stay on your path and tighten up your recovery behaviors. Soon you will know. Memories, thoughts, and feelings from the past will rise to the surface when you are ready to know and to remember.

Exercises: Deepening My Growth in Early Recovery

Craving and Impulse

Remember the craving, the life-and-death urgency of grabbing for something? You had this impulse during your active addiction and you have it in new recovery. But now it is quiet. Now, most of the time, you are not driven by painful need, fear, or anxiety. You can slow down; you can stop and think. You can reflect.

- Do you remember the intensity of new recovery? Do you remember your drive to act, your need for quick help and quick answers? What is it like now?

_____

_____

_____

_____

Safety and Stability

- Can you describe a time when you felt calm and safe? A time when you knew you had recovery tools and you used them? What was it like to feel this new security in your recovery?

_____

_____

_____

_____

- List five tools you use to feel calm and stable in recovery.

_____

_____

_____

_____

Recovery Learning

Once you are anchored in recovery, you can focus on your growth. That means focusing on reality and widening the breadth and depth of your world, both past and present. Like a young school child, you will be learning new words and a new language to tell the truth about you. You will build your "story," that is, the reality of who you were, what you did, and who you are now.

- What was it like for you to learn new words of recovery? What was it like to speak this new language—to realize that you had phrases, that you were no longer a raw beginner? What is it like now to live, breathe, and speak recovery? Does the language of recovery feel natural or still foreign?

- When did you tell your story for the first time? What was it like? How did you feel?

- Did your story change as you progressed in early recovery? If yes, how did it change? If no, what did change for you as you moved into early recovery?

- When did you first look outward, toward others, from the vantage point of a woman in recovery? How did you feel? Has your view of others changed?

  _____

  _____

  _____

  _____

- What major issues and hurdles have you encountered in early recovery? Make a list with two columns: "Self" and "Other Relationships." (Or use the chart below.) List the key issues, themes, or hurdles you have explored. Let these lists grow, adding to or changing them as you progress in recovery.*

SELF	OTHER RELATIONSHIPS
Behavior	*Behavior*
Old Behavior:	Old Behavior:
New Behavior:	New Behavior:
Head Learning	*Head Learning*
Old Ideas:	Old Ideas:
New Ideas:	New Ideas:
Conflicting Ideas:	Conflicting Ideas:

* This exercise may be part of your Fourth and Tenth Steps.

Heart Learning	Heart Learning
Old Feelings:	Old Feelings:
a. Negative:	a. Negative:
b. Positive:	b. Positive:
New Feelings:	New Feelings:
a. Negative:	a. Negative:
b. Positive:	b. Positive:
Conflicting Feelings:	Conflicting Feelings:

Staying on the Path

• How do you stay on the recovery path? What is your daily program? What recovery actions do you take? What do you think about? What is your recovery focus? What do you feel? How do you maintain your anchor in recovery?

_____

_____

_____

_____

_____

Recovery and Trauma

Early recovery is the time when memories of trauma may slowly surface. Or they may push and prod at you to get to work. You may have sudden flashbacks—memories from the past—that intrude full force into your wide-awake daytime world or your nighttime world of dreams. When it is time to deal with the traumas of your life, begin slowly. You have a lifetime to remember all that haunts you. However, you may have to intensify the pace of your work on trauma if you have trouble maintaining your sobriety.

If you get too scared, too anxious, or too depressed, you may feel a wavering in your program. If you start to wander away from your anchors of recovery—and wander into detours of false excitement, distraction, and denial—you may put your recovery at risk. Then you must go back to the basics of your program, recommit, and seek professional help. It is normal to feel conflict in recovery. It is normal to feel frightened of what you might see or know. So try not to withdraw too far. You can take all the time-outs you need, but hold on to your recovery base.

Below we are going to continue looking at the trauma-related questions that were discussed in chapters 2 and 3.

- How was your addiction traumatic for you?

- What has been traumatic in recovery? Have you felt overwhelmed or have you lost control?

- What traumas have you experienced in your life?

_____

_____

_____

_____

_____

Relapse

You may have returned to drinking or using other drugs after you began recovery. Or, you may have feared relapse as you maintained your recovery.

- If you relapsed, what happened to you? When did you go back to drinking/using? Do you understand why and how it happened?

_____

_____

_____

_____

_____

- How did you get back to recovery?

_____

_____

_____

_____

_____

- What do you do to maintain recovery? Write a description of your relapse prevention program.

What Is Real?

- As you remember back to your active addiction, and as you think about what it was like to lose control, ask now, what does *real* mean for you today? What do you know absolutely? What is true?

What Is the Gift?

- You have been through the past, you have remembered and you have accepted what is real. What is your gift today? What do you know about yourself or your recovery that you couldn't recognize before? What are the gifts of seeing and knowing once again? Name some forgotten interests that you are reconnecting with.

Chapter Five

Grown Up and Living Sober

THE ONGOING RECOVERY STAGE

You are now a grown-up in recovery. Does this mean you are "fixed"? Is your healing process finished? The answer to both of these questions is "no." Being a grown-up means you can now rely on your recovery. Recovery is who you are, through and through. You have a sense of competence deep within you, born of your hard work. You own the principles of recovery, and recovery behavior is automatic, though you still pay attention to old instincts and pulls from the past. You are fluent in your recovery language and you know the depth of feelings, past and present, within you.

Maintaining and Deepening Your Recovery

In the ongoing recovery stage you bring your healthy self to everyday life. You stay open and honest, ready to deal with whatever comes. You deepen and expand your relationship to your self, to others, and to your Higher Power. This deepening is held by your trust in the process, your growing capacity to be honest, and your increasing ability now to let go.

Remember your false self? Remember that cocoon of defense that so defined you during your active addiction? You were full of denial, but you didn't see it. You believed you had control, or you wished you could control anybody or anything. You could never understand "letting go," and maybe you thought you didn't need to. In ongoing recovery you look at yourself and that whole issue of control. You look at how you acted in relationships. You now have a better sense of what "give and take" means in a relationship. You can tolerate an unfolding, open-ended exchange. You can engage in dialogue—conversations that go back and forth—that you don't need to control or withdraw from.

Letting Go of Defense as a Way of Life

Our old defenses don't go away over night. Maybe you thought they would disappear forever, along with your character defects. It is good to remember that as much as our psychological defenses used to do us in, they also protected us. We will have defenses to recognize and deal with forever just like we will see remnants of our character defects throughout our lives. We don't grow into perfect people. We grow into people who are *more* honest, open, genuine, humble, accepting, generous, and forgiving.

Maybe you used to feel very self-important. You had a big dose of grandiosity; you had no limits. Grandiosity is an important defense for people who don't think they're very important at all. It is like adding Teflon to that cardboard bunker of your false self. In ongoing recovery, however, you have uncovered your old, false self in the Fourth Step and you keep it in check by continuing to work all of the Steps.

You still may rely on projection, that convenient way of disowning what really belongs to you. Projection is the attribution to someone of a thought or feeling in the self. For example, you are sure that your husband is upset with you, so you lash out at him in anger. In ongoing recovery you quickly focus on yourself and you chuckle when you realize these unwelcome thoughts or feelings really belong to you. You now can see that instead of your husband being upset with you, you are upset with him.

Rationalization may still be one of your fall-back coping skills, but you no longer let it entirely drown out your better judgment. Now you recognize your rationalization and ask yourself, "Do I really need to make these excuses for my poor behaviors?"

In ongoing recovery, you get to show up for you. You get to see yourself, watch your defenses closely, challenge them when necessary, and settle into acceptance of who you are. You are real, genuine, honest, and open. You do not need to live behind a false self of defense.

Expansion of Self

With stable, ongoing recovery, you get to grow bigger and wider and deeper. When you were actively addicted, you lived in a narrow inner prison. You were small inside and growing smaller. Now you feel an ever-expanding space within. You will feel more, see more, and know more about yourself. At the same time you also realize that you know less and less. You have come to trust "not knowing." It doesn't scare you. And so you will take emotional risks. You may find a new depth of grief and sorrow. You may even experience the grief of acceptance. You can grieve who you were and what happened. You can grieve what you did not and could not know—then and now.

You will feel happiness and sorrow, love and hate, anger and understanding. You will feel more of everything as your inner world grows larger and you feel safer.

Sometimes women in ongoing recovery experience what we call a "second recovery." Suddenly, something is wrong. A woman feels afraid, she's depressed, too sad for too long, and she has no idea what is the matter. Hopefully she stays solid on her recovery path. She delves into deeper emotional work. Perhaps she has traumas from the past that now surface. She knows now that "something wrong" could also signal that she is doing "something right." She has more work to do and now she trusts that she can do it.

As she lives in ongoing recovery, she may ask, "Who am I now?" She is a woman long separated from her active addiction who has a healthy dependence on her recovery program, friends, and mentors. She has found the boundaries of her "self," and she now knows clearly where she stops and others begin. And she has a bigger capacity for feeling, seeing, and knowing. She is held safely by her deep belief and trust in her Higher Power.

Expansion of Self and Other

In early recovery you began to look outward and question how you operate in relationships. Being honest with yourself is not easy, but learning to be healthy in a good relationship will keep you busy forever more. Your first close relationships in recovery may be with other recovering women, including your sponsor. These were your first experiences of healthy dependence in relationships. Now you know what interdependence is. Now you know what real intimacy is. Getting to this point hasn't been easy, and it won't be easy now. Close relationships can be difficult, but you now choose to work hard at them. You have a growing capacity for empathy. You can deeply understand another. You can be separate and independent, separate and interdependent, and you can be separate and dependent too. You don't need another person to make you whole.

You learn to deepen your work in recovery and to be in close, intimate relationships at the same time. Hard? Yes. Doable? Yes.

You learn to tolerate fluidity in relationships. You live with the absence of absolutes. You have few binding rules, except you don't drink or use. And you may see these rules now as choices.

You can now feel vulnerable in relationships. This is truly amazing. You know you have come a long way. You are secure in your self and in your commitment to your sobriety. You are not selling out to someone else's need for you. You are not about to give up your healthy self. Are there challenges now? Absolutely. You face whatever life brings: riches and poverty, sickness and health, joy and sorrow. You live a sober, healthy life. You deepen and strengthen your program and live through the ups and downs. You remember the definition of healthy dependence that you learned early on: *You take care of you, I take care of me, and we support each other.* Now you know that this works because you are supported by your ultimate dependence on your Higher Power.

Relapse

Relapse can be a continuing threat. Do women relapse in ongoing recovery? Yes, but not as often as in the early recovery stage. It helps to remember the recovery axiom: *Is the pain*

I'm feeling a warning of relapse or a part of normal growth? You tighten up your recovery program until you find out—until you are given the "wisdom to know the difference." You have learned to be patient. Rarely do you act suddenly on impulse. You now can tolerate uncomfortable feelings and work through them. Ultimately, you have learned to nurture a sense of inner peace.

Despite all this growth, women in ongoing recovery can fall into the trap of not asking for help when they need it. They are now "seniors" in recovery; that is, they advise, mentor, and sponsor other recovering women. They become less open to new feelings and new learning. Ironically they begin to shut down again because they believe they should be perfect. They stop being open and vulnerable. This is a path to "arrested development" in recovery. And it is certainly a path toward relapse. The woman who thinks she is supposed to know it all needs to ask for help.

Exercises: Living Sober with My Self and Others in Ongoing Recovery

Being a Grown-up

You are now a grown-up in solid recovery. That means you have a healthy sense of self. You feel competent, secure, humble, and grateful. You know that you don't have all the answers and, ironically, this wisdom keeps you humble and open-minded. You laugh when you think about your imperfections and your pleasure in being one among many. You have a real sense of who you are—all the positives and the negatives—and you embrace them all. Your growing relationship to your Higher Power brings you security and hope.

- What does it mean to you to be a grown-up? Describe what you used to think it meant to be a healthy adult, then describe what you think a healthy adult is now. Make a list of words that describe a grown-up woman in recovery. Who is she? Who are you now?

- What are your basic principles of recovery? Think about the slogans, the Twelve Steps, or the words of wisdom you routinely rely on.

_____

_____

_____

_____

_____

_____

Maintaining and Deepening Recovery

You have a growing capacity for self-honesty and insight. You feel more, see more, and know more about yourself and your relationships. You deepen your recovery by maintaining your program and staying open to learn from the foundation of your new life principles.

- What is your daily program of recovery? What do you do to maintain your stability and to deepen your growth? Make two columns: "Maintaining Recovery" and "Deepening Recovery." (Or use the chart below.) Think about who you are and what you do in your ongoing recovery life, then list the items. Change your descriptions as you continue to grow.

	Maintaining Recovery	Deepening Recovery
Behaviors		
Thoughts		
Feelings		

	Maintaining Recovery	Deepening Recovery
Relationships		
Spirituality/ Higher Power		

Letting Go of Defenses as a Way of Life

Our defenses are very much part of being human. Can you accept all of you, even as you work to see ever more quickly when you are being needlessly defensive? We will never be free of all defenses. But, as we mature in ongoing recovery, we need the protection of defenses less and less in order to be open, honest, and secure. We recognize our defensiveness and let go more easily. That old false self of addiction now rarely nudges out your healthy self.

Defenses can be both healthy and unhealthy. Some examples of defenses include a tendency to be grandiose, sarcastic, or hot-tempered. Perhaps you use humor in a mean-spirited way. In recovery we no longer need to let defenses overwhelm our true selves. We need never be that shell of defensive cardboard that represented our false self.

- Think about defenses. What are your most commonly used defenses and how do they work for you? What situations are most likely to make you feel defensive now? What defenses keep you protected from yourself and what defenses do you rely on in your relationships? Use the chart below for your list.

Defense	How It Works for Me	How It Hurts Me

Expansion of Self

In ongoing recovery, as you come to know yourself better, you begin to tolerate and accept much more complexity about your life and relationships. You work your program to deepen your understanding of your self: who you were throughout your life, including your active addiction days and years, and who you are now. You really do understand that you haven't gone from bad to good, but you surely have gone from false to real. You get it. You know that being real is not easy. As so many women in recovery say, "You may even come to love your character defects." Ongoing recovery allows us to embrace our contradictions, conflicts, and complexities.

- Who are you now? Write down words that describe being a grown-up. What words best describe you now? What are the positives and what are the negatives? How do you feel about yourself now? What do you do to deepen your understanding of yourself?

- Have you experienced a "second recovery"? If yes, what happened? Describe how you got there and what it was like. How did you maintain your strong recovery and deepen your inner work?

- Continue to explore the trauma questions from chapters 2, 3, and 4. How is trauma, from the past or present, a part of your ongoing recovery work?

_____

_____

_____

_____

_____

_____

_____

Expansion of Self and Other

Ongoing recovery is the time for deepening your relationships. You strengthen your capacity for intimacy and deepen relationships that are not dependent on your need for control. This is not easy, but you get better and better at holding on to your self and engaging deeply with others. This happens because you have built a strong bond of dependence and trust in your Higher Power. And nobody else can do that job for you.

- How do you feel about relationships? What are the continuing struggles you face in your closest relationships? What holds you back? What keeps you closed? How do you tolerate feeling vulnerable? How do you stay safe? Write a paragraph or two about who you are in relationships.

_____

_____

_____

_____

_____

_____

- Take time to think about your recovery history and the growth of your relationship with your Higher Power. Describe your relationship with your Higher Power. What is it and how does it work for you? Trace the growth of your trust in your Higher Power. What strengthens your trust and what shakes it up?

_____

_____

_____

_____

_____

_____

_____

Relapse

Let's take a look at relapse in ongoing recovery. Yes, it still means a return to drinking or using other drugs or whatever out-of-control behavior defined your addiction. And yes, it is still possible to return to active addiction. Or you can develop a new addiction. That is why you work to maintain and deepen your recovery growth. You do not want to settle into "arrested development." You want your recovery program to hold you and guide you through all of what normal life brings.

- Have you relapsed in your recovery? What happened? How do you understand your relapse now?

_____

_____

_____

_____

_____

- What active steps do you take to maintain your recovery? If you can't tell whether your experience is a warning of relapse or part of normal growth, what do you do? Write a list of the major principles you follow to ensure that your recovery is solid.

What Is Real?

- Once again, remember back to your active addiction, think about what it was like to lose control and ask now, what does *real* mean for you today? What do you know absolutely? What is true? What is real today?

What Is the Gift?

You have been through the past, you have remembered, and you have accepted what is real. You have worked the Steps through early recovery and you have developed a strong program of ongoing recovery.

- What is your gift today? What can you feel, see, or know about you or your recovery that you couldn't recognize before? Or, what is it that you feel deeply and strongly again right now? What is your gift of seeing and knowing once again?

_____

_____

_____

_____

_____

_____

PART THREE

The Paradoxes of Recovery

Paradox is at the heart of all the major changes that women experience in recovery. A paradox turns logic upside down. The dictionary says a paradox is a statement that seems opposed to common sense, yet is true. A paradox is something with seemingly contradictory qualities that somehow work. Simply, a paradox is "not what you think it is." At first blush, it doesn't make logical sense; it feels mysterious. But when you look more deeply, it's true.

Understanding the nature of paradox is critical to maintaining a healthy process of recovery. Without paradox, virtually everyone entering recovery would feel like they had failed. Without paradox, there would be no way of turning that "failure" around, no way to grasp that the worst failure could be, and would be, the foundation of healthy growth. Without paradox, it would be very difficult to see the hard and painful work of recovery as positive. It would be hard to deeply understand the freedom granted by being one among many, of being just like everybody else. Accepting one's humanity, with the reality of human limits, is indeed the core of freedom.

Recovery is a shock of radical change, a turnaround in everything. But it is not the kind of change you expected. As you hit bottom and recognized your loss of control, as you let it be real and true, you made your entry into a new world of self-discovery and healthy growth. You came to believe "I am an alcoholic/addict; I have lost control." On this premise of utter failure of control, you formed a new attachment to recovery, a new identity as an alcoholic/addict, and new beliefs, behaviors, and feelings.

Paradox usually involves a sense of surprise. Recovery also offers continual surprises as you gain new awareness and meaning. You will also discover that, while the Twelve Steps do provide a map of the recovery path, they don't tell you what you will discover on your journey of finding your self.

In part 3 of this workbook, we will look at four major paradoxes that are part of normal recovery growth. They are also, quite simply, part of being human. Yet they are also mysterious, difficult to understand, and they sometimes show up directly as a challenge for the woman in recovery. The enduring nature of these paradoxes means that recovery growth never ends. There is always something paradoxical to explore, understand, and accept, but it often comes in or as a new shape, a new question, or a new insight. The four major paradoxes we will cover are: (1) the power in powerlessness, (2) the wholeness of a divided self, (3) independence built on dependence, and (4) relying on others although you're responsible for yourself (the apprentice model of learning in AA).

Exercises: Thinking about the Paradoxes of Recovery

- How do you define paradox?

- How does paradox work in your recovery?

- What has been the most important paradox for you in your recovery so far? Why?

ꝏ *Chapter Six* ಲ

The Power in Powerlessness

We briefly discussed powerlessness in the first chapter as loss of control—the fundamental, deep experience of helplessness. You could not stop drinking, using other addictive substances, eating, or shopping no matter how hard you tried. No matter how deeply you resolved to give it up, to get control, it didn't happen. Then you came to really see that you couldn't stop, that you were powerless to will yourself into control. And you saw and knew that your powerlessness was total and permanent. You were not going to suddenly regain control. You were not going to be able to tighten your will power or figure out the trick to getting control. Your powerlessness was deep and lasting. At that point you may have wondered what in the world could be good about this. But then, over time in recovery, you found out what was so good.

Now we look more closely at this baffling paradox: of how powerlessness can be a good thing for women. Powerlessness is at the core of addiction, loss of control, and the helplessness of being traumatized. Powerlessness is also at the core paradox of recovery: A woman's acceptance that she is powerless is the cornerstone of her healthy growth. Recognizing and accepting that she is powerless is an acceptance of having limits. It is fundamental to being human.

Yet many people never face this deep truth. They strive for self-power, self-will, and self-control. As one woman said, "I was full of self-power and I was out of control. No problem. No contradiction." Yet, all these kinds of self-power are false. They stem from an aggressive drive to gain power over people and circumstances. Nobody has this much power over themselves or anyone else. But people think they do, or think they should.

So where is the power in powerlessness? What is it? Here comes the paradox: It is the recognition of limits that holds the power for women. And the recognition of limits is precisely the deep awareness and acceptance of loss of control, the recognition of their inability—their powerlessness—to will themselves into control. Many women, especially since the birth of the women's movement, might say that accepting powerlessness is selling themselves short. They ask, "Shouldn't we strive for power, just like men? Isn't this what the women's movement was, and is, all about? Don't men have the power, and isn't this what women want?"

The struggle for social, economic, and political power is not the same as facing an addictive illness. Addiction ultimately steals a woman's power and her ability to make good choices for herself and her family. Ultimately a woman must come to face herself and to see, deeply, that she has lost control. Again, we face a paradox. As she relinquishes her belief in control, she will gain power from within.

Many women fight this recognition of powerlessness because it reminds them of past disappointments and challenges. This will be especially true for women who experienced trauma. Seeing their loss of control simply reinforces the reality of their sense of failure. They feel they have failed to be good wives, good partners, good mothers, good workers, or good people. And, as the victims of others, they may believe they must have been the cause.

An addicted woman will usually double and triple her efforts to regain control. She will make promises, commitments, and swear to get it together. But it doesn't happen. This repetitive process of digging her own grave is the core of her sense of powerlessness. Paradoxically, when she comes to recognize her role in this process she touches on her first tools for survival and healthy growth.

It is only by coming to see that she is powerless that she also comes to find her real self. When she faces her loss of control, she also says, "I am an alcoholic/addict." That "I" of ownership may be her first statement of self, and her first connection to her self. Her deep belief in her powerlessness will become the anchor of her new, recovering self. It will be the anchor of her healthy growth in recovery. It will be the deep truth that lets her reach out to others, and to accept her dependence and her need for help.

In recovery, a woman will gain a *power of capacity*, allowing her to be honest with herself and others, to know her self, and to take action. As she accepts responsibility for herself, she also finds her separateness and, shockingly, her boundaries. Seeing where she ends and another begins, and feeling her separateness, gives her power. She now can live as an active, responsible adult, acting on her own behalf. Powerlessness is the cornerstone of her self—alone. And it will be the cornerstone of the self she finds in relation to others and her Higher Power.

Exercises: Finding the Power in Powerlessness

The Experience of Powerlessness

As we have discussed, powerlessness is the loss of control and the core of addiction. Yet, while a woman is actively drinking or using, she will not recognize her powerlessness. Or, at least, she will work very hard not to see it.

- Can you remember feeling powerless when you were actively addicted? What was it like? Describe your experience of being powerless and out of control. What was it really like? If it is hard to write a narrative, just list words that come to mind as you think of the actual experience of being out of control. You may not have a clear sentence or paragraph, as these words may come like bullets, spilling out to describe your loss of control.

- When you were drinking or engaging in other addictive behaviors, what did you tell yourself was happening? How did you explain that you hadn't lost control? What was your "story"? How did you *deny* your loss of control, and *explain why* you hadn't lost control, so that you could *maintain* your addiction?

- What did powerlessness mean to you then? What did it mean to you if you thought you might be an alcoholic/addict?

Power

If loss of control is powerlessness, and this is a good thing, what is *power*? Perhaps it was connected to your idea of success. Maybe you believed that a woman's power was her self-control. You believed that you shouldn't need anything, that denial of your self was the power you wanted. What did *power* mean to you when you were actively addicted? This can be a tricky question: How could you have defined *power* back then, when you weren't supposed to have a self? What was power? For many women, power and success equaled total selflessness. Power rested in your denial that you needed anything or anybody.

- What did *power* mean to you when you were actively addicted?

_____

_____

_____

_____

_____

- What did you think about the women's movement of the mid- and late twentieth century? Did your political and social beliefs cause you confusion in thinking about your addictive behaviors? Did you fight extra hard against recognizing your powerlessness over your addiction?

_____

_____

_____

_____

- What do you think about power today? Can you find the power for you in powerlessness? How? What is it?

_____

_____

_____

_____

Limits

Many people believe that power means "no limits." To be powerful means to have end-less possibility, strength, and endurance. Power means the ability to control yourself and others. The key to the paradox of powerlessness lies in the recognition of limits. It is the experience of hitting a wall, or a definable point of "enough." When a woman comes to accept her loss of control, she gains the freedom to find her self.

- When you were actively addicted, what did you think of limits? Did you have any? What did the idea of limits mean to you then?

  _____

  _____

  _____

  _____

- What does the concept of limits mean to you now? Is it a source of power for you in recovery? How?

  _____

  _____

  _____

  _____

The Trauma of Powerlessness

As we have discussed, trauma can occur as the result of physical, sexual, or emotional abuse, through battery, and through controlling domination. Trauma can also be self-inflicted. As we have learned, an addicted woman has no choice, after a certain point, but to keep feeding her addiction. She becomes her own perpetrator, her own witness, and her own victim.

The paradox of powerlessness can be extremely difficult for a woman to comprehend if she has been the victim of another. It is very difficult for her to see that her own addiction is her responsibility. That she, in fact, can stop the addictive cycle by surrendering and saying, "I give up."

Many women in recovery have been the victim of another's harm. They may struggle mightily to accept deeply the totality of their powerlessness as a foundation for the growth of a healthy self. This woman will continually sort out what she was, and is, responsible for and what she was not responsible for. The "wisdom to know the difference" will be critically important for her healthy recovery.

Review the trauma questions from the previous chapters. *Easy does it* is good advice here. Remembering can be difficult. Many women find that sharing their memories with another (a close recovery friend, sponsor, or therapist) can ease the pain. Still, this kind of remembering can be so upsetting that it is a good idea to take it in very small doses. Keep your recovery actions and supports close by, so you can turn directly from active remembering and writing to a recovery action.

- If you feel ready, explore your past experiences of trauma. Try to focus on powerlessness. Can you remember "what it was like"? Do you have the feelings now? Can you write about your feelings and memories of losing control? If a narrative doesn't come, just let the words come out that describe your feelings of loss of control.

- If you feel ready, write about your experiences of traumatic helplessness growing up. What was it like? What happened? And what is it like for you now?

- Write about your own helplessness. What was it like to be powerless over your drinking or your other addictions? Let the words come. What was it like? What happened? What is it like now to be powerless?

_____

_____

_____

_____

Power Now

You understand the paradox of powerlessness now, or at least you get it most of the time about most things. Now you know that powerlessness can be the source of deep personal knowledge. You may also have found a Higher Power that gives you all the strength, endurance, and power that you need. Now, you have power through accepting your limits. It is no longer *self-power* or *power-over*. You discover the power of humility through relinquishing the power of self.

- What is your power now? Think about the new strengths you have in recovery. Do you have a bigger capacity—for self, for honesty, for showing up? Go back to your lists of defenses from chapter 5 and see what works as a strength for you now.

_____

_____

_____

_____

What Is Real?

- As you think about paradox, and especially about the paradox of powerlessness, what is real? What shines through today as clear? Or, what muddles you up because today it's confusing? Paradox can shine brightly or muddy the water. Feeling confusion can be as real and true as clarity. Simply think about what you know, what you believe, and what keeps you in recovery.

What Is the Gift?

You have worked hard to think about paradox, to face your powerlessness, to remember how awful it used to be and how good it is now. You have thought a lot about trauma, and you have felt it all. You know what it is to be powerless.

- How is powerlessness a gift for you?

- And, perhaps more broadly, what is your gift today? What can you feel, see, or know about you or your recovery that you couldn't recognize before? Or, what is it that you feel deeply and strongly again right now? What is your gift of seeing and knowing once again?

Chapter Seven

The Wholeness of a Divided Self

ACCEPTING CONFLICT

All people experience conflict. Conflict is part of being human. When we are conflicted, we hold opposite feelings about a person or situation. We may feel both love and hate for the same person, for example. Conflict also means ambivalence—leaning this way part of the time, and pulling back the other way the rest of the time. Conflict can cause us to feel so paralyzed about making a decision that we simply do nothing. If you are feeling paralyzed about making a decision, it is a good sign that you are conflicted.

Conflict can be conscious or unconscious. You may be aware of your mixed feelings or you may deny all your opposing wishes, wants, and feelings. Conflict can be internal—just about you and just within you. That is what addiction comes down to in the end. It is all about your life and your relationship with yourself. Conflict naturally arises when you defend your addiction, as you ignore your healthier self while the people around you often complain about your drinking, drugging, or other compulsive habits.

Internal and interpersonal conflict are universal. Accepting and dealing with conflict are particularly difficult for women who believe that they should be selfless and focus on the needs of others. They believe they should not feel conflict, and if they do, they should get over it. Feeling conflict, however, does send an important signal to a woman. Feeling conflict tells a woman that she does have wishes, wants, and needs.

Many women cope with conflict by creating a secret self, the buried real self, who holds the truths. This woman works to silence that nasty voice within that might proclaim her feelings, wishes, and wants. She may create a false self for the public while she hides her private, needy, real self.

Women are particularly prone to unresolvable conflicts because of their multiple roles and the recent changes in women's careers and social-political status. What it means to be a woman has changed radically in the last thirty years. Women are now entitled to a public, visible existence. They are entitled to have a self and a voice to speak their views. Yet this changing recognition has intensified many old conflicts for women and created new ones. Who is to be "first" in a woman's world— her self, or others? How does she define herself and how does she reconcile the multiple options that exist for her?

Women may readily turn to addiction as a solution to intolerable stress and pain. Being addicted quiets the opposition within. It softens the edges for a while and then it makes everything worse. But being in recovery may heighten a woman's conflict. Now she knows it is there and now she feels it.

Kinds of Conflict

What kinds of conflicts do women experience? Throughout history, women defined themselves by their roles, primarily as caretakers. They existed to give to others. If a woman recognized her self, she held it in secret. This double life of public and private often created conflicts, but they weren't acknowledged socially or personally. Now, women are defining themselves as separate from their traditional caretaking roles.

Many women feel a tremendous conflict between what they believe is an "ideal" woman and what they find is "real" for them. If the ideal had been to be selfless, a woman is going to struggle a lot just to recognize that she exists, that she has needs and feelings. Making her private self conscious and public is a big part of being in recovery.

A woman may fear her negative traits and feelings—those she had during her active addiction and those she still faces in recovery. She is not ideal. She is real. Seeing the reality of her deeply mixed and conflicted self just proves that she is bad—she was bad before and she is bad now. The healthy woman in recovery reminds herself that she is neither bad nor good. She is real. Conflict is real and it is normal.

In recovery, women may think that feeling conflict is a character defect. Furthermore, as they work the Steps and they see themselves more clearly, they run head on into deep internal conflict. They may feel dependent on others, yet angry about feeling needy. They may feel envy toward successful friends, yet they also feel admiration for the strength and loyalty of these same friends. It may feel like pure hate and love at the same time.

Many women in early recovery are afraid of facing their failures. But they may also fear their inner strength and power. Many women fear recovery because they sense the power they will find in speaking up for themselves.

The layers of conflict are complex. As caretakers and caregivers for the world, most women also believe that anything that goes wrong is all their fault. Addiction gave them a time-out from feeling so responsible for others and such guilt for failing. They fear that recovery will confirm that they have indeed failed and that everything is, indeed, all their fault.

But they also fear that they are not to blame for everything that goes wrong. For many women, it is easier to continue to take the blame than to face the reality that others have a part to play. This recognition can launch a woman in recovery into the difficult work of developing new kinds of interpersonal relationships.

The Path to the Real Self

A woman in recovery accepts conflict. She comes to see, know, and feel the opposition within. And she can see, know, and feel the opposing struggles she creates with others. She can see herself clearly. But getting here is not easy. She works hard on all the Steps. She works hard to deepen her self-exploration. She learns to tolerate different levels of conflict.

Trauma and Internal Conflict

A woman who has experienced trauma at the hands of others will need to face some specific conflicts in recovery. How does she reconcile what she was, and is, responsible for? How does she grapple with what was her "part" in all that happened to her? She may question what she "owes" another. She may feel nothing but confusion as she thinks about what were and are her choices. These difficult and confusing issues of responsibility will become clearer in recovery.

The Call of Multiple Roles

A woman in recovery needs to sort out who she is in relation to others. Now she can identify herself as an alcoholic/addict, a woman who lost control and who is responsible for her recovery. She may also see herself clearly as a codependent, someone who has sacrificed herself to the power of another. She may identify as the adult child of an alcoholic/addict, the adult child of trauma. She sees herself as a mother, a daughter, a worker, a wife, a partner, a runner, a teacher. She sees herself in many roles, all secondary to the core sense of her self, a woman in recovery.

Exercises: Deepening My Understanding of Conflict

What Is Conflict?

We have discussed the variety of ways a woman can feel conflicted. Now let's sort through some of your specific issues and ways of dealing with conflict.

- Did you feel internal conflicts when you were actively addicted? What sorts of feelings, needs, wishes, beliefs, or behaviors created the most difficulties for you? The most mixed feelings in you?

_____

_____

_____

_____

_____

- List five internal conflicts you struggled with during your active addiction. How did being addicted help you or hinder you in dealing with these internal conflicts?

_____

_____

_____

_____

_____

- Do you have more awareness in recovery about the internal conflicts you experienced during your active addiction? Can you see the past more clearly? Do you experience the same conflicts now?

_____

_____

_____

_____

_____

• List five internal conflicts you understand and struggle with in recovery. How has being in recovery helped you or hindered you in accepting and dealing with these internal conflicts?

• Did you feel interpersonal conflicts when you were actively addicted? What sorts of feelings, needs, wishes, beliefs, or behaviors created the most difficulties for you? The most mixed feelings in you?

• List five interpersonal conflicts you struggled with during your active addiction. How did being addicted help you or hinder you in dealing with these interpersonal conflicts?

- Do you have more awareness in recovery about the interpersonal conflicts you struggled with during your active addiction? Can you see the past more clearly? Do you have the same conflicts now?

_____

_____

_____

_____

- List five interpersonal conflicts you understand and struggle with in recovery. How has being in recovery helped you or hindered you in dealing with these interpersonal conflicts?

_____

_____

_____

_____

- Because your understanding of conflict may change over time, and because the kinds of conflict you felt during your active addiction and the kinds of conflict you feel now may change, you might find it helpful to use the chart below to keep a record of conflict. What were your conflicts then? What are your conflicts now? You can add to or change your lists as you deepen your recovery. Happily, you may also see many conflicts soften, or even resolve, as you grow healthy in recovery.

	Internal Conflict	Conflicts with Others
During Addiction		
In Recovery		

Kinds of Conflict

A woman feels all kinds of conflicts. One is simply the pain that comes from denying that she has a self and feeling the truth of her self deep within. Then comes the pain of seeing and accepting that she does have a self. She may feel guilt and failure for existing. She may also feel terrible guilt and failure because she has failed to live up to her ideal of being self-less and in control. What a shock to find that she has a self—"I am an alcoholic/addict"—and to see that her sense of self is built on loss of control.

A woman in recovery changes her ideal. She does that by being in recovery. What is real—who she is—becomes more acceptable and more healthy to her and, hopefully, to others. She may fear seeing anything negative about herself, yet she knows that the negatives are there. Yes, she is angry; yes, she is needy; yes, she is ambitious; yes, she wants her independence, but she doesn't want to feel alone. On and on it will go—coming to see these normal struggles of conflict.

- Use the chart below to deepen your understanding of conflicts you experience. You may find that these exercises fit in especially with your Fourth and Tenth Steps. Use the examples to get you going.

EXAMPLE
Kinds of Conflicts

	What is it?	What's the conflict?
My beliefs	I should be able to make everyone happy.	I can't take care of me and make everyone happy at the same time.
My values	I value deep honesty.	I'm afraid to be honest with people because I'll disappoint them.
My feelings	I often feel sad and angry.	I'm supposed to feel happy and cheerful.
My needs	I need to feel emotionally safe with others.	I'm afraid of others. I can't trust anyone.
My wishes	I secretly long to be taken care of.	I know I'm supposed to be responsible for myself.

Kinds of Conflicts

	What is it?	What's the conflict?
My beliefs		
My values		
My feelings		
My needs		
My wishes		

The Path to the Real Self

Staying on the recovery path can be especially hard for women who feel intense conflict. It is crucial to learn to recognize conflict and to accept the opposing pulls within.

- How do you deal with conflict? What is your program of self-exploration to understand conflict? How do you stay on the path when you cannot resolve the internal strife or contradictions within?

Trauma and Internal Conflict

How do you sort through the traumas of your life? How do you recognize childhood trauma and then understand the conflicts that resulted for you? This is not easy. This is part of the long work of ongoing recovery. You may want to work with a therapist to remember and deal with the realities of your life. Again, you may have to face yourself as a victim of another, and as a victim of yourself, your own loss of control to your addiction. Take it slowly. Do seek help doing this work.

- If you feel ready, how do you think about trauma? What does it mean to you? What can you see now about the traumas of your life? Start with a simple memory and add images and words as they come. Remember, you do not have to solve painful memories or conflicts that resulted from your traumatic experiences. You just need to know them.

The Call of Multiple Roles

You always had multiple roles and you have multiple roles now. In the chart below, list your past roles (from when you were actively addicted) and your current roles (now that you are sober). Where is your deepest experience of self in relation to your roles?

MY ROLES	
Then	**Now**

What Is Real?

- As you think about conflict, maybe you are much clearer than you have ever been about what your issues are. Perhaps you are even more confused. Think about what is real today. What do you know absolutely? What is true today? Meditate for a few minutes on these questions and write a few comments. What is true today for you?

_____

_____

_____

_____

_____

_____

What Is the Gift?

You have been immersed in thinking about conflict. You have accepted that it is normal, and now you know you've got it! You have seen that you struggle with mixed feelings, wishes, needs, behaviors, and beliefs about lots of things. You struggle inside, in relation to yourself, and you struggle with others.

- What is good about conflict? Does it feel like your acceptance of conflict is a gift? What is your gift right now? Or, what is it that you feel deeply and strongly again? What is your gift of seeing and knowing once again?

_____

_____

_____

_____

_____

Chapter Eight

Independence Built on Dependence

BECOMING SEPARATE THROUGH CONNECTION

Most people believe that dependence is a bad thing. They think they should be self-sufficient and never rely on others. This is, of course, impossible. Dependence is part of human nature. Instead of trying to do away with dependence, we need to redefine it. Healthy dependence is important to human growth and human relationships. On the other hand, unhealthy dependence, like addiction, arrests human growth and impairs human relationships.

Most people, men and women, fall somewhere in between feeling completely independent and completely dependent on others. They match an American stereotype: an ideal of self-sufficiency (tough, macho, frontier strength) paired with an underlying, often hidden, desire to be taken care of. Women have carried an impossible double bind. Until recently, they were supposed to be strong as the nurturing caretakers of their families, yet they were not supposed to be so strong that they could be self-sufficient. Women learned: Be strong for others and have no needs yourself. Of course women did have needs. They met them through their caretaking of others, and secretly, through all varieties of self-soothing, including self-medication. They felt guilty for having a self, for recognizing their abilities, needs, and desires. To this day, many women believe that they are selfish if they think about themselves.

This entrenched cultural view of women has changed dramatically during the last fifty years, though these deep beliefs remain. Many women still define themselves *only* as caretakers of others. They have difficulty identifying their own needs, wants, and wishes separate from others. This makes it difficult for women to find a middle ground between independence and dependence, that midpoint of mutual dependence. The long, hard work of recovery helps a woman find her new definition of independence: an acceptance that she is dependent on others and that she stands alone. She manages these seemingly opposite truths through mutual human dependence with an ultimate dependence on her Higher Power.

The Dependence in Independence

Dependence and independence are not separate categories. You are not one or the other, despite your deepest beliefs. If you are alive, you are dependent. No one can survive without others. A healthy, gratifying dependency on parents and other caregivers during infancy and childhood will lead to both a strong sense of self—autonomy—and a strong sense of *self-with-other*. This self-with-other concept refers to a capacity for relatedness based on mutual dependence, or interdependence, on others.

Unhealthy Dependence

This healthy interaction between self and self-with-other is difficult for Americans to grasp. Americans seem to expect people to jump from infantile dependence to self-sufficiency in a simple leap. This can force people to deny their genuine needs. This denial of need is a core feature of addiction. Women can end up denying that they have any needs at all, while they meet their needs through the use of substances, including food, and other behaviors that give them the illusion of self-sufficiency. This denial of need turns into a secret addictive cycle. The denial of dependence as a human need turns into unhealthy dependence.

Women and men need others, not just in infancy. Healthy dependence throughout life is *the* key to healthy growth and a healthy self. Yet accepting dependency remains difficult as long as it is equated with weakness, disempowerment, and inequality. The great paradox for a woman in recovery rests on these three ideas, all related to dependency:

1. A woman must openly acknowledge that she exists, that she has a self.
2. She has needs and has been meeting these needs through her addiction.
3. She is both dependent on others and autonomously responsible for herself.

Many women readily accept their dependence. They have trouble acknowledging a self and then accepting their ability to act on their own behalf and take care of themselves. These women will often adopt a trade-off: "I deny my self and ability to take care of my life; I exist to take care of you, and I expect you to take care of me in return." The result for many women is disappointment and an unhealthy path to addictive "self-care."

What Is Independence?

As you will surely know by now, independence is not total self-sufficiency. Nor is it pseudo-independence, a pretense of total self-sufficiency (looking strong and self-sufficient to the outside world while secretly harboring and meeting your intense hunger, cravings, and needs). Independence is not a denial of need. Independence is autonomy, a deep experience of being separate from all others, of existing alone, yet also connected with others. Healthy independence is an acceptance of personal freedom, the separateness from all others, along with an acceptance of need and self-responsibility. A woman in recovery grows into healthy independence by accepting her dependence and experiencing a new, healthy dependence that will give her a sense of inner strength. She grows into her freedom by knowing her limits. She accepts that she is an alcoholic/addict and that she needs help. This is her deepest experience of knowing that she is helpless, out of control, and that she cannot get control. She cannot survive alone.

She comes into recovery by asking for help. She reaches out to establish a new attachment, just like an infant reaches out to its mother. She reaches out to other women in recovery and to the principles of recovery, usually through AA or another Twelve Step program. She trades her unhealthy dependence on her substance for a new, healthy dependence on the people of AA.

She will now discover mutual dependence. She finds the paradox of "alone and alone-together." She learns that the women of AA can support her, but they can't do it for her. They can't relieve her cravings or stop her from drinking or using. Her feelings and her behaviors are hers alone. She can take action on her own behalf as she relies on others to show her how they did it and to offer her support. She will learn that healthy independence is based on healthy dependence. It is the result of being engaged in a new process of development. The woman in recovery faces herself alone as she connects with others.

Spirituality

A woman in recovery learns about spirituality through experience. Developing a sense of spirituality takes time for many women in recovery. It is difficult to realize that addictive substances and behaviors became like a "Higher Power" that left her entirely dependent. Now, as she accepts her human need, her loss of control, and her deep human limits, she comes to find a healthy dependence. Early on in recovery, this dependence will be on other women and the new principles she is learning. Later in recovery, she will find a "Higher Other," which she will likely call her Higher Power.

Trauma and Independence

We are now going to revisit the dilemma of trauma and dependence. As discussed earlier, the addicted woman is a victim of herself. She may also have been the victim of others. Either way, she is not likely to have a deep trust in dependence on others. No way. She may be OK with the idea of autonomy, but she would like to get it without having to accept her dependency. And so, she may have a "resistance to recovery."

For many women, relationships of dependency have hurt. Lack of power in relationships is all they have ever known. So why should they trust anyone? To counter their traumatic experiences in close relationships, women may develop a sense of self-sufficiency that is not based on pseudo-independence or a false sense of strength. It is based on a deep need for protection. They do not feel strong; they feel weak, helpless, and vulnerable. They believe at their core that other people will hurt them. These women survived by withdrawing into themselves to avoid an emotional connection with others. How then can they possibly trade their dependence on a substance for a reliance on others?

This trading of dependencies will be at the heart of a long, slow growth in recovery. Daily interactions include an "old me" alongside a "new me." Women learn a new kind of dependence, a trust in the greater power of AA and their own Higher Power, which they come to define. Being dependent through connection is not a loss of self. It is a claim of self. No one takes over for you. Others show you and you do the work. You develop a new meaning of trust: "You take care of you and I take care of me and we support each other."

Exercises: Deepening My Understanding of Dependence and Independence

What Is Dependence?

- It is time to explore how dependency affected your life. How did you think about dependence when you were actively addicted? What did dependency mean to you?

- How did you feel about dependence when you were actively addicted? How did you feel about your own dependence—the cravings and need that you knew you had, but perhaps denied?

- What was your "dependence of choice"? Your drug of choice? Your addiction? What were your other unhealthy dependencies? List five unhealthy dependencies and describe how they were unhealthy.

- How do you think about dependence now? What does it mean to you?

- How do you feel about dependence now? What are your healthy dependencies?

- List five healthy dependencies and describe how they are healthy now.

What Is the Dependence in Independence? What Is Mutual Interdependence?

Being dependent or independent is full of paradox. First of all, independence is not self-sufficiency. It is not what people would like to think it is. Dependence need not be a total loss of self, which people fear. There is no such thing as independence without healthy dependence. But integrating both concepts of being dependent and independent into one concept—rather than being one or the other—is incredibly difficult to grasp. You grow into a healthy integration that becomes mutual interdependence.

Being independent is autonomy, an acceptance of self that comes through accepting self-responsibility. The road to this kind of healthy autonomy begins with a healthy dependence. It is the foundation for healthy infant and child development and the foundation for healthy growth in recovery. Yet it is terribly difficult to understand. Most women who enter recovery have an abhorrence of dependence. They don't want it. They don't know what autonomy is and they are frightened to find out.

- What did you think about dependence and independence when you were actively addicted? Did you have a sense of both? Did you have a sense of what healthy dependence is? Of what independence is? What did autonomy mean to you?

- What do you think about dependence and independence now? Do you have a sense of both? Do you have a sense of what healthy dependence is? Of what independence is? What does autonomy mean to you now?

- What is mutual interdependence? Write a paragraph about what it is and how you have come to know it. Describe how mutual interdependence works for you now.

_____

_____

_____

_____

_____

What Is Spirituality?

Many recovering women develop a profound sense of spirituality. This often is rooted in their deepening understanding that they alone are responsible for their addiction. They learn to rely on other people for support, but they come to see that their deepening belief in a Higher Power will guide them into being a person who is responsible, interdependent, and autonomous.

- How did you think about spirituality when you were actively addicted? What did spirituality mean to you then? Did you think about spirituality as dependence?

_____

_____

_____

_____

- How do you think about spirituality now? What does spirituality mean to you? Do you think about spirituality as dependence?

_____

_____

_____

_____

Trauma and Independence

Every addicted woman knows how traumatic it is to be totally out of control and not be able to stop using. Many addicted women also know how traumatic it is to feel helpless in an abusive relationship with a spouse or partner. Trusting one's self and others can be a long, slow process. As we have done in other chapters, let's think about you and trauma. Again, these are tough questions. Take your time and do get help. Be sure you always have a recovery action ready to follow your self-exploration. Some of these questions will be part of your Eighth and Ninth Steps. Some of them may come up right away in Step One as you struggle to accept and remember being powerless.

- How do you think about you, your addiction, and trauma? Can you see that you were out of control? How does it feel to you now? Can you see that your addiction was a dependence that kept you out of control?

- List the ways you were out of control besides your addiction. Did you think or act self-destructively in other ways? Perhaps hardest of all, were you harmful to others?

- While growing up or during your active addiction, were you the victim of others? What happened? How were you helpless in relation to another? Can you remember feeling out of control?

- List the ways in which you were out of control as a partner in a traumatic relationship. How were you self-destructive to maintain a relationship? How were you harmful to others?

What Is Real?

You have been immersed in the paradoxes of dependence and independence. You have a good grasp of what mutual dependence is. You know that you are autonomous, you are responsible for yourself, and that you need others too. You know that you are ultimately dependent on your Higher Power to hold you alone and alone-together.

- Think about what is real for you in this moment. What is real today? What is the one thing you know for sure? What is the one thing that is certain and that keeps you sober?

What Is the Gift?

Again we get to think about the gifts. Here you are full of awareness of your needs and desires, of your freedom and responsibility, and your real, true sense of interdependence. It works for you. You have opened the door to trauma and perhaps you have gone deep down. Maybe that exploration is ahead of you. No matter where you are with dependence and independence, with a trust in others or your Higher Power, think about your gifts today.

- What recovery gifts are you experiencing right now? What do you feel deeply and strongly again? What is your gift of seeing and knowing once again?

Standing Alone with the Help of Others

THE APPRENTICE MODEL OF AA AND OTHER TWELVE STEP GROUPS

By now you know that there are many keys to healthy growth in recovery and they are all paradoxical. Everything seems to be backward, even though it's not. One of the paradoxes you now know by having lived it in your own recovery is the importance of connection. You have an understanding that you will come to better know yourself by being open to others, and by allowing them to show you their recovery path. You begin to understand that you will find your separate, healthy recovery self *through* your relationship with others.

You learn to rely on others while being responsible for yourself. You learn from others so that you can stand alone. It seems crazy at first: How can you exist alone, really alone, and be connected with others at the same time?

Wanting Someone to Take Over

So often, when a woman thinks of needing help, she thinks of it as all-or-nothing. She may expect to be rescued, hoping that someone will swoop in and take her away from her self-destructiveness. She may long for such a rescue, but she may also fear it. She is certain there is a price to pay for rescue: the loss of herself to someone else's authority. She wants to be taken care of, yet she wants to be in charge of herself—and the two desires don't seem compatible. This can be a major conflict.

Some women may scoff at the idea that they need or want any help at all. They take care of themselves and they have done it forever. This woman stands alone without the help of others, without the connection to learn from others. She believes it is all up to her. This woman may also feel conflict. She would like to be open to asking for help, to recognizing her need for help, but she cannot allow herself to think positively of others. As a child, she may have experienced terrible trauma at the hands of others, perhaps from her parents or others responsible for her care, and she cannot trust that anyone would be able to help her. Help always meant harm. Help always meant manipulation, a high price to pay.

A woman in healthy recovery will come to experience a place in the middle, where she can rely on herself but comfortably find support in others. As she matures in recovery, she will strengthen her connection with her Higher Power who becomes her strongest "other."

You may have heard about the apprentice model of AA; this refers to how we learn from others so that we can stand on our own. This is the paradox: *alone-together.* When a woman observes how others take care of themselves in recovery, she learns how to do that for herself. As she sees how others accept responsibility for themselves, she learns to nurture this in herself.

What Is the Apprentice Model of AA?

Apprenticeship involves more than watching. It also involves an emotional attachment to recovery—to the meetings, to the symbols of recovery (such as the books and medallions), to the people who model their recovery, and to a Higher Power. This attachment will be the dependency relationship that provides the early and ongoing security of new development, the base for new learning, for growing up all over again.

A woman in recovery also learns by doing. Taking new action is central to being in recovery and to internalizing the new growth. You learn to substitute recovery behavior and thinking for addicted behavior and thinking. You learn these new behaviors and thinking by watching, listening, and maintaining your emotional attachment to recovery.

A woman in recovery learns to trust others whose primary focus is to take care of themselves. She learns to depend on them to keep their focus on their own recoveries. Only then can she trust that she can focus on herself too. She learns that she can't find recovery in isolation, she can't find recovery totally from within. If she only looks inside, she will find her false self, the woman who became addicted and lost her true self. She confronts the paradox that she has to look outside of herself first, to look to others who have come before her, as the path to finding her new self. She looks to others to show her the way and then she shows it to another. This reciprocal learning and teaching is ongoing and often indirect. The apprenticeship experience is always present in the structure of AA—in the meetings, in the readings, in work with a sponsor, and in work with others. The source of learning exists in the ongoing interdependence that is central to AA.

How Does It All Work Together?

Moving from isolation to connection can seem overwhelming. You may have coped with emotional pain and conflict as you tried to listen to others, but felt shame in your sense of need. Or, you couldn't stop wishing that someone would just work the recovery program for you. It was just too painful to recognize that the responsibility would end up with you.

By being in recovery, you have learned to "talk the talk." You have your own story now, and it keeps growing as you develop a bigger capacity to be honest with yourself and others. You are fluent in the language of AA, and it has a depth of meaning for you because you "walk the walk." You live with a deep acceptance of your need for others and your responsibility for yourself.

The Parts of a Twelve Step Program

The developmental model of recovery is based on membership in a Twelve Step program. It is this membership, this emotional attachment to recovery, that allows for the fundamental move from isolation to connection, from reliance on self-alone to self-with-other. The woman in recovery will find the "other" by being in a meeting, reading, writing, listening to and watching others, and usually by having a sponsor. The sponsor is the mentor, the one who teaches directly by her own example, and by direct instruction. As people in AA say, the sponsor shares her own "experience, strength, and hope" with her sponsee.

Relationships with sponsors can be easy or difficult, smooth or rocky, or usually, some of both. The woman in recovery will soon learn that her sponsor cannot be her Higher Power. Nor is the sponsor a replacement for mother or father, or for what was always missing. But the sponsor may nevertheless be motherly or fatherly and may indeed offer a great deal by example that will help the sponsee fill in holes of development.

Relationships with sponsors and with peers in AA can be full of ups and downs. They are likely to remind the woman in recovery of her lifelong experiences with others, for better and worse. As she grows in recovery, she can use her experiences with others to look more deeply within to examine her deepest wishes, needs, and conflicts and to see herself more clearly—again, for better and worse.

Higher Power

A woman's growth in recovery is ultimately held and guided by her belief in, and attachment to, a Higher Power. She may not start recovery with a belief in a Power greater than herself. Indeed, for many women, their addiction was their Higher Power, the highest "other" they ever knew. As a woman deepens her development of self, through learning from others, she will also deepen her sense of a Power greater than herself, and greater than any other person. She will strengthen her dependence on her Higher Power, which she has constructed for herself in recovery, and this dependence will allow her to feel, and to be, equal with all others. She can then flourish in the apprenticeship relationship— everyone is equal, everyone learns from others, and everyone passes it on.

Transformation

The woman in recovery is not the same woman she was when she was drinking or using or consumed by her loss of control. She is no longer focused on trying to get control. She is not longing to find the power in her self, though she may sometimes wistfully long for the delusion of self-control when reality is hard.

The woman in recovery has experienced a transformation, precisely by relinquishing her belief in her own power and coming to believe in a Power greater than herself. She has also been transformed through her experience of connection with others. She does not stop growing. She does not reach the end of recovery. She does not ever find self-sufficiency, and she is not looking for it. She comes into a sense of her healthy self by acknowledging her dependence, her limits to power, and her need for others, all held by a belief in a Higher Power. She accepts responsibility for herself and she relies on others to show her what responsibility is and how to claim it.

Exercises: Standing Alone with the Help of Others: Learning to Learn from Others

What Is Connection?

Connection is a key to a healthy self. This is one of the great paradoxes of recovery. Connection with others in recovery and with a Higher Power is what allows a woman to find her self. Connection lets her know that she is alone and that she is responsible for herself. Connection lets her live with a deep awareness of her self alone and alone-together.

This paradoxical understanding can be hard to grasp. At first a woman may believe that connection will spare her from finding her self. She may wish that someone would take over and rescue her from herself. Or she may fear connection. She may not want anything to do with anybody else. Isolation and her false belief in self-sufficiency may be her only security.

- What did you think about connection when you were actively addicted? What did it mean to you?

_____

_____

_____

_____

• What did you think about other people when you were actively addicted? What did you think about relationships? How did you feel about people and how did you feel about relationships?

• What does *connection* mean to you now? What does it mean to you in relation to other people? What does it mean to you in relation to your Higher Power?

• How does connection work for you in finding your self?

Asking for Help and the Apprentice Model of AA

Asking for help is usually difficult for women. Asking for help has been an all-or-nothing proposition. You either wanted someone to take over and do it for you or you wanted no part of anyone else. So now you learn that asking for help in recovery is a key to finding and growing your healthy self. It is indeed hard to make sense of this. So many women struggle in recovery to find the experience of interdependence, the meaning of this middle ground of asking for help and giving help. They learn how to be on the receiving end of help as a new woman in recovery, learning from others who have come before. And they learn how to "pass it on," sharing their own experience, strength, and hope with others. Asking for help in recovery automatically becomes reciprocal. Learning to learn from others is a circle. That is the healthy connection.

- What was it like for you to ask for help when you were actively addicted? What were your attitudes, beliefs, and feelings about asking for help? How did you feel about the people you asked for help?

- What was it like for you to ask for help when you were a child? Do you have specific memories of times you asked for help? What happened? What was it like? How did these experiences shape your feelings about needing help or asking for help? What impact do your past experiences have on you today?

- Draw a large circle of connection. Draw smaller circles within the larger circle to illustrate your relationships with others. Include a circle, inside or outside, for your Higher Power. There is no right way to do this exercise. It simply serves as a picture of you and your mutual interdependent relationships.

- Fill in the following blanks with the names of people, objects, tasks, or exercises—whatever it is that you rely on and trust to help you. For example, you might write: "I depend on meetings to give me support in staying sober." Write as many dependencies as you can think of. Put this exercise away and come back to it another time. Add, subtract. Look inward to see how you feel about these dependencies. What feels OK? What is hard?

  I depend on _____ to _____.

  I depend on _____ to _____.

  I depend on _____ to _____.

- Fill in the following blanks with the names of people, objects, tasks, or exercises—whatever or whomever it is that depends on you. For example, you might write, "The people in my Sunday meeting depend on me to have refreshments ready at the start of the meeting." Write as many dependencies as you can think of. Put this exercise away and come back to it another time. Add, subtract. Look inward to see how you feel about these dependencies. What feels OK? What is hard?

  _____ depends on me for _____.

  _____ depends on me for _____.

  _____ depends on me for _____.

- How did you feel about the idea of learning to learn from others when you were still actively addicted? How do you feel about this idea now? Write a few sentences or more about what it means to you to learn from others and to have others learn from you.

- What is *interdependence* for you? What does it mean and how does it work?

How Does It All Work Together?

Being a healthy woman in recovery is a step-by-step process. First, the woman forms an attachment to recovery and perhaps to people in recovery. Then she begins to learn from these others. At the same time she is learning, someone else will be learning from her. This process takes her from very small beginning steps of behavior change to deeper learning. She begins to think differently about herself and her addiction. She begins to know herself and she begins to feel. She remembers her past and she comes into her new, healthy sense of self in the present.

This process occurs *through* her connections with others and with her Higher Power.

• Think about how this apprenticeship process occurred for you. Begin to write a story about your recovery, just like you have the story of your addiction. What happened? How have you learned to be in recovery? How have you learned about yourself?

_____

_____

_____

_____

_____

_____

• What advice do you give to others about being in recovery? Do you have key points that are most important to you in your recovery process? How do you pass it on?

_____

_____

_____

_____

_____

_____

The Parts of a Twelve Step Program

All Twelve Step programs have a similar structure. And while meetings vary, they all bring people in recovery together and all involve some degree of sharing of experience. Individual members take turns in holding service positions. Members share a commitment to "carry the message" to alcoholics and addicts who are still suffering.

All of these elements come together as a model of apprentice learning. You learn from others and you take responsibility for yourself. All of these elements and the experience of being part of something larger than oneself bring connection. For many, it is the first experience of feeling "part of" something while maintaining a healthy sense of self.

- How do you think about your Twelve Step program? How do you feel about your involvement? How does it work for you?

_____

_____

_____

_____

_____

_____

- Fill in the blanks:
  a. This is what I love about my Twelve Step program:

  _____

  _____

  _____

  _____

  b. This is hard for me in my Twelve Step program:

  _____

  _____

  _____

  _____

- Have your Twelve Step meetings, or the people in your Twelve Step world, ever reminded you of your family? Have you struggled at different times with this difficult experience? With the feelings that are opened within and the memories that come? Write about your experience of the past being awakened in a Twelve Step setting. Just like dealing with trauma, this can be a difficult and painful exercise. It can also be very helpful. If it is too hard, put it aside or work with your sponsor or a friend. Always consider consulting with a therapist if the emotional work of recovery is blocking your growth.

_____

_____

_____

_____

_____

_____

Higher Power

The concept of a Higher Power is part of Twelve Step recovery, and it is unique and particular to every single person. There is no single Higher Power for you to accept or reject. A huge part of your recovery work is developing a belief in a Higher Power, or returning to a belief in a Higher Power you had lost a connection to.

- What was your Higher Power when you were actively addicted? What is your Higher Power now? This may not be something you can easily describe, and it may feel too limiting to write about it. You may simply want to write down words that come to your mind that remind you of your Higher Power, or words that give you a connection.

_____

_____

_____

_____

_____

Transformation

When a woman stops drinking or using and enters recovery she may experience a sudden sense of transformation. For others, this sense of transformation takes place over a long period of time as they accept responsibility for themselves and learn to connect with others. They are transformed by a growing sense of healthy self and self-with-other. It is a long, hard road to this wondrous place of transformation, but it is always worth it.

- How do you think about transformation? How do you feel about it? Can you describe the transformation(s) you have experienced? What happened? How? What do you tell others about change?

_____

_____

_____

_____

_____

What Is Real?

Here we are at the end of the paradoxes. Whew, what a long hard road. Grasping the complexities of your life and the complexities of change is hard. But here you are, becoming "one among many" and truly experiencing interdependence. You have looked at what it means to ask for help, to learn from others, and to pass it on. You have looked inward, as you now do routinely, to see what you think and feel about this new experience of connection. Now it is time once again to pause and ask simply, "What is real today?"

- What do you know above all else to be real for you today? What is it and why is it important?

_____

_____

_____

_____

_____

What Is the Gift?

And here we are again looking for the gifts in recovery. What do you know today—absolutely—that is your gift? What is it that you have been given, that you have received? What have you allowed to be yours, coming from "other."

- What is your gift right now? What do you feel deeply and strongly again? What is your gift of seeing and knowing once again?

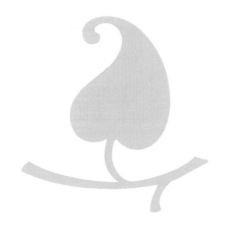

PART FOUR

At Home in Recovery

✺ Chapter Ten ✺

The Gifts of Recovery

Awoman in recovery gets what she wants, but not in the way, shape, or form she expected. A woman in recovery has a new self she could not have envisioned and could not have set out to construct by herself. Her new self is the *result* of her commitment to recovery and her engagement in a long developmental process. Women speak of many gifts, including the ability to have goals and aspirations, to experience desire and intent, and to go after what they want. Women feel a sense of mastery and competence born of experiencing a healthy self. Women feel strength and stamina, born of self-acceptance. They also accept emotion and experience a sense of belonging and a new-found feeling of self-respect. The mature woman in recovery has a healthy self. That is the promise of recovery for women. Growing into a new, healthy self is the transformation.

Goals and Aspirations

You are in recovery and you now own your right to a separate self. You also own your responsibility to continue growing. You began your recovery development by acknowledging to yourself that you are an alcoholic/addict. That was the beginning. Perhaps all you wanted then was to feel better. All you could dream of was the end of cravings, the end of shaking. And then, as days and weeks passed, you felt better. The cravings receded and the shaking stopped. You could begin to grow in recovery through your new abstinent behaviors, working the Steps, and using the help and example of others.

Now you are in ongoing recovery. You have done the hard, often deeply painful work of digging and remembering and stepping up to claim your responsibility. Now you know who you are, and you can allow yourself to feel your wishes. Now you can have desires, goals, and aspirations, and you can pursue them.

This is a huge gift for most women and it is not easily claimed. Many women continue to fear their own wishes long into recovery. It was always taboo to think about yourself,

99

or it was dangerous—someone would object if she had her own wishes and needs, or if she were successful.

But healthy recovery gives you the opportunity to acknowledge your self. You begin to sort through what you want, allowing yourself to move toward your new goals: goals that are born of your recovery growth, goals that are now realistic and achievable because you are in recovery.

You know that you can have goals, and you know that you cannot control the outcome. You can work, step by step, to achieve what you want, and you know that you have limits. The pursuit of your goals and aspirations may stretch you, but your solid, stable ongoing recovery program holds you. You now know risk and reward—always within limits.

A Sense of Mastery

Mastery is a feeling of internal security and trust, a competence born and grown from within. It has nothing to do with "getting control." Attempts to "get control"—of yourself or others—come from the head, from the will, from a sense of exercising "power over." Mastery is born from the relinquishment of this drive for will and power. You get mastery when you stop fighting for control, seek help, and begin to learn from others. This is what happens when you recognize that you are an alcoholic/addict and you surrender to the reality of your loss of control. Then you ask for help and the process of recovery development begins. Remember, you are just like the child who grows up with a healthy attachment to healthy parents. The child will learn from her parents who she is and how needs are met. The woman in recovery has the same opportunity.

Strength and Stamina

You have a new kind of strength. It is not physical strength or the strength of will. This is inner strength, born from your long work of recovery and your relationship with your Higher Power. Inner strength is not "power over." It is true empowerment, an experience of inner strength that you grow into. Stamina is part of it. Stamina is not "holding on for dear life." Rather, stamina is an inner wisdom that helps you hang in for the hard work and let go when you need to.

Both strength and stamina are the direct result, the gift, of a partnership with your Higher Power. You know how to work your program to find the balance between a focus on yourself, your recovery, and your relationships with others. Your inner strength is born of your deep belief in the ongoing rightness of your world as you stay deeply attached and committed to your recovery. You feel calm within, most of the time, as you trust you will have the strength you need, when you need it.

Accepting Emotion

When you were still drinking or using you may have expressed your emotions in harmful ways. Perhaps you tended to be quick-tempered. Or perhaps you kept all your emotions under tight wraps. In new sobriety perhaps you felt the dam burst and it may have scared you to death. Would all the crying ever stop?

Sometimes in new recovery, you feel numb and you are relieved to live without feeling. Slowly but surely, however, as you progress in your recovery, the feelings will come. You won't welcome them at first, but, eventually, you will be glad to know that you can feel. You will have feelings about the past and the present. You will feel sad and glad, sorry and forgiving, grief and joy, and everything else.

As you grow in recovery, your inner world of feelings grows too—bigger, wider, deeper. You become a richer woman because you can now feel so much more, and you don't think there is something wrong with you because you feel. You have learned to watch the feelings arise within, to name them, and to let them be inside of you. Maybe you express them, maybe you don't. You know what they are and whose they are.

Belonging

So many women struggle with the notion of belonging. Am I a part of this family/group/community? Do I want to be a part of this family/group/community?

How can I fix myself so that I will belong? How can I feel OK about myself when I don't want to belong, when I see myself standing apart? Back and forth, in and out, is how it often goes.

Oh, what conflicts. The woman in recovery will almost certainly get to face this issue in some form. She may resist joining a Twelve Step group because she fears what that will mean. Does she want to be an alcoholic/addict among other alcoholic/addicted women? Not likely, before she's sober. Has she always been an outsider and proud of it? For many women, belonging is too frightening. It means a loss of self, even a false self. Women may struggle for years with how to belong to AA and not belong at the same time.

Some women jump right in. They feel right at home and they know they belong. It's just not a big issue for them. They may have some trouble when it comes to figuring out what it is they want, separate from others. They may not know how to stand alone.

Despite all these conflicts, most women come to know a deep sense of belonging. They grow into this feeling and knowledge, just like they grow into all the other gifts. They discover that belonging has a new meaning when they know that they also stand alone, that they are responsible for themselves. Then belonging means the interdependence of healthy sobriety.

Respect for Self

You have found self-acceptance. You know how you feel and what you want, even if it takes you time to figure it out. You can stand by your own wishes, feelings, thoughts, and desires. You no longer have to craft yourself to be somebody else's ideal. You are you and that is the woman you bring to the world.

You grow into this self-respect, just like you grow into everything else. It is often hard, especially early on, to hang on to what you know and believe in. But you will get there. You will be able to make hard choices and to know that they are the right ones for you. You will be able to hold on to yourself and to compromise with others. You exist as a woman alone, and alone-together. You learn that yielding does not mean a loss of your self. Self-respect is the gift of finding your self and growing your self into the healthy woman you want to be.

A Healthy Self

Well, here you are. You have grown into your healthy self by engaging in a process of recovery. What does it all mean? You laugh when you tell your story. How can it be that you are powerless to the core, full of conflict, dependent, and deeply grateful for your sober self? How can it be that you have come to find your self through this rugged road of hard work? How can it be that "selfishness" has brought you here, the key to finding your healthy self? It is all about paradox, which you now understand. That is why you laugh. Sometimes you cry too. It is hard. But, oh is it worth it! You feel blessed and grateful. You have been committed to your recovery, to accepting responsibility for yourself, and you have learned to learn from others. You know that every day you have a choice and every day you choose for your recovery.

Exercises: The Gifts of Recovery

What Are the Gifts?

As a woman grows into her healthy self in recovery, she will experience many gifts. These are changes in her, new ways of seeing her self and others, and new strengths she finds within herself. They are gifts because they are the *result* of being in recovery. These are not changes that she could will or force. These are, most of all, not changes that are based on successfully taking control. No. All of these gifts have come from surrender, asking for help, and accepting responsibility for herself. They are all the results of living in paradox.

- What are the gifts of your sobriety? What do you think of immediately? Make a list and let the words flow. Keep writing and then come back and write some more. Your gifts are your own.

- Next, think of why the items you wrote above are gifts. See if you find paradox. Are these gifts you never could have imagined?

Goals and Aspirations

Many women in healthy recovery can have goals and aspirations, a gift that comes with finding a healthy self. You know that you want, and you know how to figure out what you want. It is now OK to have desire. It is OK to look ahead and to plan. It is OK to reach for what you want. You can meet your goals and aspirations because you know how to ask for help, how to work step by step, and you know your limits.

- Think back to the beginning of your recovery. Did you have goals and aspirations then? What were they? What did you allow yourself to hope for?

- Was it hard for you to have goals? Did you feel conflict as you thought about what you wanted? What were these conflicts?

_____

_____

_____

_____

_____

_____

- How did your goals and aspirations change as you progressed in your recovery? Do you remember a time when you felt OK about your desires and wishes? Can you remember what they were as you strengthened your recovery? Do you remember milestones?

_____

_____

_____

_____

_____

_____

Mastery

Perhaps you had a sense of mastery as a child. Perhaps you knew the sense of competence that came from within you as you learned to ride a two-wheeler, as you learned to add and subtract and then to divide and multiply. That feeling of "getting it," of feeling capable, is what mastery is. At the beginning of recovery you may feel like a total wreck. You may learn that you shouldn't trust your own judgment because look what happened. As you become stable in recovery you may have your first taste of mastery and it's a wonder. You know how to be in touch with someone. You know what to do if you need help. Later on, you will feel mastery about many other things as you grow into your healthy, real self.

- What does mastery mean to you? List five experiences of mastery you had when you were first sober. What was it like to feel competent about something in recovery?

_____

_____

_____

_____

- Now list experiences of mastery you have now. Write all you want and add to this list as you grow in your recovery.

_____

_____

_____

_____

Strength and Stamina

Strength and stamina come from within. You grow into this deep sense of knowing, of calm, of trust that you will survive. You trust in your capacity to endure, as you work the Steps and engage in the developmental process of recovery. Strength and stamina are gifts of your healthy relationship with yourself and with your Higher Power.

- Think back to when you were first sober. Did you feel any strength and stamina then? What did you feel about your inner self and your capacity to face recovery?

_____

_____

_____

_____

- Think about your strength and stamina now. How do you feel strong? What does *inner strength* mean to you? What does *stamina* mean?

_____

_____

_____

_____

_____

_____

_____

Accepting Emotion

Emotion is part of recovery for every woman, but each woman has her own particular relationship to her feelings. Some women feel a lot of emotions early on in recovery. Some can't feel at all for a long time in recovery, while others wax and wane. They feel a lot and then they don't feel. They go through an intense period, perhaps stimulated by Step work, or by sudden memories of trauma that surface. No matter when you feel, how much you feel, or what you feel, you will be able to have a deeper experience of your emotional self, free from alcohol and other substances. This is a great gift, though it may be hard to accept. The woman in recovery welcomes her feelings and works to understand them. She knows they are a vital part of her healthy self.

- When you were first sober, did you have feelings? What were they? What did you think about them? If you didn't have feelings, what did you think about that?

_____

_____

_____

_____

_____

_____

- How have your feelings expanded in recovery? How have they deepened and widened? Do you have a "story" of the birth and growth of your emotional self?

- Write a list of feelings that come to you spontaneously. See which feelings you like and which feelings you don't like. Can you connect these feelings with any memories in recovery?

Belonging

Do you feel that you belong in recovery? Belonging in recovery is often hard won for women and full of conflicts. But as a gift of recovery, belonging is the great wonder of feeling part of something that is bigger than you. It may be a particular meeting, it may be a sense of your connection to women all over the world, or it may be that good feeling you get every time you hear a woman say "I'm an alcoholic/addict."

- What was it like for you when you went to your first AA or other Twelve Step meeting? How did you feel? Did you have a sense that you belonged, that you were in the right place? Did you have conflicts? What were they?

• Write your story of belonging. When did you feel that you belonged to your Twelve Step group? What was it like? Do you feel a sense of belonging in your life? How is belonging a gift for you?

Respect for Self

You are you and that's that. You have a deep acceptance of your self as you have grown in your recovery. You know who you are now and you bring your self—your real self—to your relationships. Through being in recovery and working the Steps, and through your relationships with others and your Higher Power, you are solid, secure, and the "right size." Respect for your self is a result of your hard work.

• What did *self-respect* mean to you when you were first sober? What does *self-respect* mean to you now?

• Write all the ways you respect your self and keep this list open, like others you have begun. As you grow in your experience of self-respect, write a note about what happened and how you felt.

A Healthy Self

Here you are, at the end of this workbook, but not at the end of your recovery growth. That goes on. By now, you probably have a sense of your own healthy self. You know where you've been and where you've come to, and you've got a sense of how to do it. You know recovery, and you know that your attachment to recovery and your continuing engagement will hold you steady and healthy, no matter what happens. You know paradox. You know that your journey of recovery began with calamity, with your surrender to your loss of control. You learned that powerlessness was freedom and the core of your new growth in recovery. You learned that you need others but you also stand alone, and you learned to learn from others to be able to take responsibility for yourself.

Healthy recovery is a great gift, a gift you have worked hard for.

- Now it is time for your recovery story. Who are you now? Write the story of you, a healthy woman in recovery. Take time and return to this story whenever you feel you have more to tell, or more to explore.

- Every day you make choices. What are your choices today?

• Think back to the end of every chapter of this workbook and the questions you
  answered. (What is real for you today? What is your gift today?) Now think
  about all the things that are real for you now and all the gifts you have
  received. Let this list grow too.

  _____

  _____

  _____

  _____

  _____

  _____

• You are a healthy woman in recovery. What would you tell a woman who is
  new to recovery about the journey ahead?

  _____

  _____

  _____

  _____

  _____

  _____

The Twelve Steps of Alcoholics Anonymous*

1. We admitted we were powerless over alcohol—that our lives had become unmanageable.
2. Came to believe that a Power greater than ourselves could restore us to sanity.
3. Made a decision to turn our will and our lives over to the care of God *as we understood Him.*
4. Made a searching and fearless moral inventory of ourselves.
5. Admitted to God, to ourselves, and to another human being the exact nature of our wrongs.
6. Were entirely ready to have God remove all these defects of character.
7. Humbly asked Him to remove our shortcomings.
8. Made a list of all persons we had harmed, and became willing to make amends to them all.
9. Made direct amends to such people wherever possible, except when to do so would injure them or others.
10. Continued to take personal inventory and when we were wrong promptly admitted it.
11. Sought through prayer and meditation to improve our conscious contact with God *as we understood Him,* praying only for knowledge of His will for us and the power to carry that out.
12. Having had a spiritual awakening as the result of these steps, we tried to carry this message to alcoholics, and to practice these principles in all our affairs.

*From *Alcoholics Anonymous,* 4th ed., published by AA World Services, Inc., New York, N.Y., 59–60.

The Twelve Traditions of Alcoholics Anonymous*

1. Our common welfare should come first; personal recovery depends upon A.A. unity.
2. For our group purpose there is but one ultimate authority—a loving God as He may express Himself in our group conscience. Our leaders are but trusted servants; they do not govern.
3. The only requirement for A.A. membership is a desire to stop drinking.
4. Each group should be autonomous except in matters affecting other groups or A.A. as a whole.
5. Each group has but one primary purpose—to carry its message to the alcoholic who still suffers.
6. An A.A. group ought never endorse, finance, or lend the A.A. name to any related facility or outside enterprise, lest problems of money, property, and prestige divert us from our primary purpose.
7. Every A.A. group ought to be fully self-supporting, declining outside contributions.
8. Alcoholics Anonymous should remain forever nonprofessional, but our service centers may employ special workers.
9. A.A., as such, ought never be organized; but we may create service boards or committees directly responsible to those they serve.
10. Alcoholics Anonymous has no opinion on outside issues; hence the A.A. name ought never be drawn into public controversy.
11. Our public relations policy is based on attraction rather than promotion; we need always maintain personal anonymity at the level of press, radio, and films.
12. Anonymity is the spiritual foundation of all our traditions, ever reminding us to place principles before personalities.

*From *Twelve Steps and Twelve Traditions*, published by AA World Services, Inc., New York, N.Y., 129–187.

About the Author

STEPHANIE BROWN, PH.D., is a pioneering researcher, clinician, author, teacher, and consultant in the addiction field. A psychologist, she is the director of the Addictions Institute in Menlo Park, California, where she also has a private practice. She is a research associate at the Mental Research Institute in Palo Alto, where she codirects the Family Recovery Research Project. Dr. Brown is the author of nine books, including the companion text for this workbook, *A Place Called Self: Women, Sobriety, and Radical Transformation.*

Hazelden Publishing and Educational Services is a division of the Hazelden Foundation, a not-for-profit organization. Since 1949, Hazelden has been a leader in promoting the dignity and treatment of people afflicted with the disease of chemical dependency.

The mission of the foundation is to improve the quality of life for individuals, families, and communities by providing a national continuum of information, education, and recovery services that are widely accessible; to advance the field through research and training; and to improve our quality and effectiveness through continuous improvement and innovation.

Stemming from that, the mission of the publishing division is to provide quality information and support to people wherever they may be in their personal journey—from education and early intervention, through treatment and recovery, to personal and spiritual growth.

Although our treatment programs do not necessarily use everything Hazelden publishes, our bibliotherapeutic materials support our mission and the Twelve Step philosophy upon which it is based. We encourage your comments and feedback.

The headquarters of the Hazelden Foundation are in Center City, Minnesota. Additional treatment facilities are located in Chicago, Illinois; Newberg, Oregon; New York, New York; Plymouth, Minnesota; and St. Paul, Minnesota. At these sites, we provide a continuum of care for men and women of all ages. Our Plymouth facility is designed specifically for youth and families.

For more information on Hazelden, please call **1-800-257-7800**. Or you may access our World Wide Web site on the Internet at **www.hazelden.org**.